BOOK DESCRIPTION

A comprehensive look into red light therapy.

Are you tired of dealing with chronic pain, inflammation, or skin conditions that just won't go away?

Do you feel like you are constantly fighting an uphill battle with your health?

Have you tried all the traditional and non-traditional treatments out there, but nothing ever seems to work?

Do you want a shot at slowing or even reversing the aging process?

Well, look no further than Red Light Therapy, the revolutionary treatment that harnesses the power of light to heal and protect every system in the body. In this comprehensive guide, we delve into the science behind red light therapy and provide you with all the information you need to understand how it works and why it's so effective.

In this book, you'll find:

· A breakdown of the different wavelengths of light used in Red Light Therapy and how they target specific health concerns

· Tips on how to optimize your Red Light Therapy sessions for maximum benefits

· A comprehensive list of common health conditions that can be effectively treated with red light therapy, including acne, eczema, and arthritis

· Everything you need to know before buying a red light therapy device

· How to calculate your own red light dosage and maintain your treatments

· How to optimize your personal treatment plan

Red Light Therapy is the best-kept secret in healthcare today, and with this book, you will have all the information you need to unlock its full potential. Whether you are a beginner or a seasoned user, this book will provide valuable insights and tips to enhance your red light therapy experience. From understanding the science behind this innovative therapy to learning about the different types of devices available, you will be equipped with the knowledge to make informed decisions about your treatment and get the desired results. Click on the "Add to Cart" button now and improve your health in ways   you   never   thought   possible.

THE COMPLETE GUIDE TO RED LIGHT THERAPY

Simple Uses for Pain Management, Anti-Aging, Fat Loss, and Cognitive Function

TABLE OF CONTENTS

References

INTRODUCTION

Light equals life. From the moment we are born, we are bathed in the warmth and radiance of light. It fuels our growth, nourishes our bodies, and even helps our brains perform at their peak. It helps us sleep, recharge, and even heal. But did you know that light at a specific wavelength can be used for so much more? In this book, we will explore the fascinating world of Red Light Therapy, a revolutionary technique that harnesses the power of specific wavelengths of light to heal, protect, and rejuvenate the body.

This book will discuss the fascinating world of red light therapy, how it works, and why it is so effective. We'll look at some of the easiest and most effective ways to use it for yourself. From the convenience of at-home devices to the options available at professional clinics, you'll discover a variety of approaches to incorporating red light therapy into your daily routine. We'll also be diving into the science behind red light therapy, exploring the specific wavelengths and frequencies that make it so powerful for healing and cellular regeneration. As a believer in the power of light, I am thrilled to be able to share this information with you. Knowledge is power, and it's time you got your hands on some special power. So, what are you waiting for? Let's get started!

CHAPTER 1: WHAT IS RED LIGHT THERAPY?

"The truth is always beautiful and simple, and it says that there is only one disease: a dysfunctional cell."

— Buckminster Fuller

Light, like nutrients from food, is required for human cells to operate properly. When a sick cell is exposed to the correct wavelength of light, it can activate its metabolism. Specific wavelengths of light can help power up our cells, impact hormones and neurotransmitters, regulate our mood, boost physical performance, speed stress recovery, promote alertness, improve sleep, and favorably affect gene expression. This may appear to be a weird thought at first since we are not accustomed to viewing light as a potent method of stimulating the body. Instead, we think of light as this mysterious, intangible force that appears to be nothing more than a benign form of illumination, but as science has proven, there is much more to light than meets the eye.

The human body is made up of billions of cells that rely on different biological processes to function properly. These cells have the ability to absorb and respond to different wavelengths of light, including red light. When we don't have enough energy or are injured, our bodies make repairs and build new cells in order to heal themselves, which is a great thing, but these repairs can lead to infection and inflammation if they go unchecked. This is where red light therapy comes in. When exposed to red light, cells repair themselves, but in a way that does not overstimulate or irritate them. This results in a safer and quicker healing process. No other type of light therapy has been as effective at treating inflammation and rejuvenating the body as red light therapy, with many people noticing results within just a few minutes of use! The human body needs light to function properly, and in this chapter, we are going to open your eyes to the absolutely astonishing ability of light to heal.

So, What Exactly Is Red Light?

Red light is the part of the electromagnetic spectrum that has a wavelength of 600-740 nanometers. The human eye can detect this specific wavelength of red light, but the wavelengths we are interested in are beyond what the human eye can detect. So how does the red light work?

The human body can create its own molecular vibration frequency. We go through life unaware of this fact because our cells don't consciously resonate at this frequency, but it is no coincidence that when people are exposed to red light, their cells start vibrating at their own natural molecular frequency. The frequency shift is so powerful that it can cause deep healing for physical and even mental health problems.

This phenomenon, known as photo-biomodulation, has been the subject of extensive research in recent years. Scientists have discovered that red light, with its longer wavelength and lower energy, has the ability to penetrate deep into our tissues and interact with our cells in profound ways. By stimulating the production of ATP, the energy currency of our cells, red light can enhance cellular metabolism and promote the regeneration of damaged tissues. This therapeutic effect of light is not new, and for thousands of years, cultures in every part of the world have used light as a form of healing. Eye-opening scientific research is now proving that light has the power to convert organic matter into energy. And this ability is precisely what gives red light its legendary healing properties.

In simple words, red light therapy is the process of exposing the tissue to red light. This therapy is also known as bio-stimulation, photo-biomodulation, or low-level light therapy (LLLT). It is used to treat a wide range of chronic health conditions, including cardiovascular disease, neurological disorders, gastrointestinal problems, pain syndromes, muscle inflammation, and issues related to bone healing. The science surrounding red light treatment is expanding on a daily basis and has made headlines with claims that it can slow or even reverse the aging process.

Scientists now know that red light therapy functions by interacting with our DNA to promote the creation of new mitochondria (the powerhouses of our cells) and increase the number of stem cells available for cellular regeneration. The increased number of stem cells that develop as a result of red light therapy can be used in the treatment of degenerative illnesses, including cancer.

Origin of Light Therapy

Light therapy has been used for thousands of years. The ancient Egyptians, Greeks, and Romans used sunlight as a source of healing, favoring it over toxic medications and invasive surgical procedures. To use particular colors of the visible spectrum to treat illness, the ancient Egyptians built sunrooms with colored glass panes that would filter the sunlight. They believed that each color had specific healing properties and could target different health issues. Similarly, the Greeks and Romans built temples dedicated to sun worship where patients would bask in the sunlight for therapeutic purposes. Many of these healing temples have been discovered by archaeologists, demonstrating that the use of light as a means of healing has been a tradition for eons.

While oil and gas-fueled lighting paved the way for illuminating the night, the invention of the electric bulb revolutionized our understanding of and ability to control light. When Thomas Edison filed the first incandescent light bulb patent in 1879, it positively transformed our ability to influence the environment. As scientists learned more and more about how light functions and interacts with our biology, the field of light therapy took shape as a viable form of treatment for disease.

Niels Ryberg Finsen, a physician from Denmark, began experimenting with light to investigate its impact on living things after Edison invented the incandescent light bulb. Dr. Niels created the first light therapy in 1896 to treat a form of TB called lupus vulgaris. He could cure a 2-cm-diameter region of damaged skin with an electric light rich in ultraviolet light. The daily, two-hour therapy sessions he had were so effective in getting rid of the disease's lesions that he went on to establish a facility where he saw 804 patients, many of whom experienced success. This remarkable use of light therapy earned Dr. Niels the Physiology Nobel Prize in 1903.

As decades flew by, interest in the therapeutic properties of light waned and was replaced by contemporary medical medication and surgical procedures—that is until the laser was invented, ushering in a new age of light therapy. The invention of the laser transformed light therapy because, from that point on, scientists were able to create highly concentrated beams of light, allowing for precise targeting and a wider range of wavelengths.

For more than 50 years, lasers have been used to treat dermatological conditions and even perform delicate eye and spinal surgeries. But it wasn't until recently that red light therapy was revived as a viable form of treatment when researchers at the University of Toronto discovered its mitochondria-stimulating properties.

How Red Light Therapy Works

DNA (deoxyribonucleic acid) is the genetic material in every cell that tells our cells how to operate. Within the DNA strands are millions of genes (small sections of DNA) that generate our cellular identity. These genes determine the way our cells operate. By influencing our DNA through the process of photo-biomodulation, red light therapy changes the way our genes function. It does this by modifying the cells' metabolism so that they operate more efficiently and effectively. As an active energy molecule, red light stimulates our mitochondria to produce ATP, the cellular life force. This heightened production of ATP increases the process of cell reproduction and creates a situation where our cells are able to function effectively. The result is improved cellular metabolism, leading to increased cellular regeneration.

As our bodies grow and develop over time, the DNA in every cell is duplicated at each cell division. This duplication process is a critical factor in cellular function but can become damaged or become too active by triggering one or more genes simultaneously. This can result in cells starting to unnecessarily replicate sequences of DNA, doubling and then tripling the workload for our mitochondria. When this happens, our cells no longer function as efficiently as they should, but red light therapy can help relieve this stress on our cells by reducing the replication of DNA through the stimulation of mitochondrial oxidase and Nrf2 pathways. In simpler words, red light therapy targets "surplus" genetic material in our cells, gets rid of it, and allows for healthy, normal cellular regeneration. By keeping our cells operating at an optimal level, we are able to maintain a high level of health and prevent many degenerative diseases.

Red Light Therapy and Mitochondria

Mitochondria are tiny, specialized structures within our cells that convert the nutrients we consume into energy. They play a pivotal role in cell health because they keep our bodies running smoothly. A healthy number of mitochondria leads to an efficient metabolism, which in turn keeps our cells happy and healthy. A decrease in the number of mitochondria is associated with disease symptoms like fatigue, pain, weight gain, and inflammation.

Mitochondria are what we call the "powerhouse" of the cell. They break down all of the nutrients we consume and convert them into energy, which our cells then utilize to produce cellular repair. By increasing our mitochondria's ability to function properly, red light therapy reduces stress on our cells and increases their lifespan.

Red light devices are made up of red LEDs that emit microwaved infrared energy. This red light penetrates the lipid bilayer surrounding our cells, making it available for use by our mitochondria. Inside the cell, this infrared light stimulates the mitochondria to produce ATP (energy) by activating the reduced nicotinamide adenine dinucleotide (NAD) oxidases. While NAD is known to exist in our cells, the activation of its oxidases results in the creation of nicotinamide adenine dinucleotide phosphate (NADPH). This NADPH helps speed up the cellular degradation processes that result in an increase in the number of mitochondria.

The mitochondria inside our cells play a critical role in cellular health and function. The movement of electrons from the mitochondrial matrix directly into the cell's cytoplasmic membrane stimulates nutrients inside of your cells and increases their functionality. Red light therapy assists this process by instructing your mitochondria to produce this energy without any complications.

The information provided by the mitochondria in a cell is directly related to the overall health of that cell. A properly functioning mitochondria will tell the cell how to operate efficiently, avoiding disease-causing cellular dysfunction and apoptosis (cell death). A mitochondrial deficiency can lead to cellular dysfunction and even cause malignant cells to multiply. Red light therapy prevents this by improving a cell's ability to utilize oxygen, which hemoglobin delivers through our bloodstream. Hemoglobin is an iron-based molecule found within red blood cells that transports oxygen to your tissues. Red light therapy improves our blood's ability to deliver oxygen by increasing the body's production of hemoglobin. This results in more efficient delivery of oxygen to all of the body's cells, including our mitochondria.

Red Light Therapy and DNA Repair

Our DNA has an important job in keeping us healthy: it determines who we are as a person. When DNA is damaged, cells can become cancerous or diseased. DNA damage is so important because every time a cell divides into two new ones, it carries with it all of the mistakes and faults that it previously experienced. For this reason, DNA damage is closely related to the aging process because the cell will repeat this cycle of mistakes, and malignant cells will be born.

Our DNA is the blueprint for how our cells function throughout our lives. It determines all our characteristics, including how we process information, make decisions, think creatively, and manage emotions. The left and right sides of our DNA are responsible for encoding this information in proteins that are then used to build the cell's protective wall. When this protection fails, we become vulnerable to disease. Failure in our DNA repair system can lead to cancerous tumors or other serious health problems. Red light therapy can help target issues with DNA so that you can avoid illness and premature aging and stay healthy as you age.

Your cells possess DNA repair mechanisms that can detect damage to your DNA. This damage can come from a number of sources, including chemicals, radiation, viruses, and hereditary factors. Our DNA is designed to repair itself when damaged, but it may not be able to do so completely if the cell has lost too many mitochondria to begin with. Red light therapy can help increase the production of mitochondrial energy so that the cell's DNA repair mechanisms can provide maximum protection to the genome. Having a properly functioning DNA repair system will result in a longer lifespan and prevent the development of diseases like heart disease and Alzheimer's.

Red Light Therapy and Telomeres

Telomeres are found at the end of each chromosome in a familiar-looking shape, like a "crown." Telomeres actually prevent DNA from fraying, protecting our genetic information after cell division. However, they are not able to repair the damage that is done to the chromosome. Our cells may stop dividing altogether when telomeres are damaged through excessive oxidation or other harmful processes. This is known as cellular senescence, and the resulting cells become old, dysfunctional, or even cancerous.

Telomere length can help us predict overall health and the risk of disease. Shortened telomeres are associated with a higher incidence of many age-related disorders, including atherosclerosis, arthritis, diabetes, and osteoporosis. Red light therapy increases your body's production of telomerase, an enzyme that processes and repairs telomeres. This increases the lifespan of your cells, preventing them from becoming old and ill and quitting replicating. Increased telomerase activity means longer telomere length, which then reduces the chances of cellular senescence and premature aging. Telomerase is also known to play an important role in the health of blood cells like red blood cells and white blood cells, which fight infection. A healthy, longer-lived blood cell population will reduce your risk of genetic diseases and other degenerative health problems.

The Ideal Wavelength for Red Light Therapy

Red light is the best wavelength to use for increasing cellular health since it can penetrate deeper into the skin, reaching more cells. The longer the wavelength, the better it can reach into your derma, reaching your blood vessels and other vital organs like your kidneys or liver. For red light therapy, the general consensus is that the wavelength should not exceed 940 nm, but many doctors run the boxes at up to 1,000 nm to get the most range for the treatment.

The exact exposure time for red light therapy will vary depending on which condition you are using it for. The exposure time is the number of minutes that it takes for red light to reach a particular place within our body. Your doctor should advise you on the length of time between treatments and how many times per day you should have them, but a dosing guide will be included in this book just in case.

What Does Red Light Therapy Treat?

When it comes to addressing disease symptoms, red light therapy is a highly effective alternative to mainstream medicine that most doctors can prescribe. It can be used to treat all of the following conditions:

1. **Pain:** Red light therapy is an excellent treatment option for those suffering from general pain. It helps to reduce acute inflammation in the body, which is often at the root of many chronic conditions like arthritis, muscle pain, and headaches.

2. **Headaches:** Headaches may be caused by inflammation, stress, or a number of other factors, like excessive caffeine consumption. Red light therapy can help reduce pain in the muscles that are responsible for your headaches by making them more relaxed.

3. **Joint Pain**: In addition to helping reduce pain from muscle strains, chronic inflammation, and headaches, red light therapy can also help provide relief from joint pain by relaxing the surrounding tissues and increasing the lubrication of your joints in between. This makes movement smoother and less painful overall.

4. **Circulation:** Red light therapy is an excellent treatment option for those suffering from poor circulation. It helps to improve blood circulation in all of the extremities, including your palms and feet. It also helps to improve circulation in the gut and lungs, making it a great option for those suffering from digestive issues, asthma, heart disease, and more.

5. **Dizziness and Vertigo**: Vertigo or dizziness can be caused by whiplash injuries or other types of injuries to the inner ear.

Red light therapy can help reduce and ease the symptoms of vertigo by relaxing your inner ear.

6. **Chronic Pain:** Chronic pain can be caused by many issues, including joint pain, arthritis, and migraines. Red light therapy can help reduce pain caused by these conditions as well as lessen the effects of other chronic conditions like fibromyalgia, which are related to inflammation.

7. **Muscle Spasms:** Muscle spasms are caused by a number of factors, including injuries, stress, and muscle fatigue. Red light therapy can help to relax the muscles in your body, which means you will start to feel less pain and stiffness even after being engaged in an activity that you once considered strenuous.

Key Takeaways

· Red light therapy is a non-invasive method of treatment that is considered by many to be an effective alternative to traditional medicine.

· The wavelengths used in red light therapy are carefully chosen to reach deep into the derma, making it effective for treating a wide variety of health conditions.

· Red light therapy is perfect for maintaining healthy cellular function and, when used correctly, can help improve the length and quality of your life.

· Red LED lights are available at the highest power possible while still remaining safe for human use.

· The potential applications for red LED lights are many, but they have yet to be fully explored. For now, people are using them to treat a wide variety of age-related illnesses and symptoms, including chronic pain, migraines, and muscle strains.

Red light therapy is still in the early stages of its development within the mainstream medical community, but it is continuing to gain traction for its ability to help reduce inflammation in patients suffering from pain and illness related to their cellular health. Red LED lights are finally receiving the attention they need to continue to be used for treating the aging population. The human body is a remarkable piece of technology and is continually evolving. But as we age, our bodies struggle to keep up with environmental stressors and push through changes we didn't anticipate or can't control. Unfortunately, this is just par for the course for most of us, but it doesn't have to be this way. With the help of red LED lights, you can take control of your health and treat the parts of your body that need healing most, including your skin, which is one of the most common places for cellular damage to occur. So, if you're ready to go deeper, the next chapter will address the confusion between near-infrared light therapy and red light therapy. Wouldn't you like to learn the real difference between the two?

CHAPTER 2: RED VS. NEAR-INFRARED LIGHT

"We are a walking bundle of frequencies tuned into the cosmos—sound and light waves that have been slowed down. We are souls wrapped in holy biological robes, and our bodies are the instruments on which our souls perform."

— Albert Einstein

Our ancestors worked in the sun and around fires for extended periods each day, both of which release a lot of red and near-infrared light, meaning that once upon a time, we were exposed to far more of the proper wavelengths of light. As a result, for hundreds of thousands of years, humans didn't need to worry about the effects of light deficiency since they were able to meet their daily demands for red and near-infrared light by living outside in the sun. Fast forward to recent generations, and contemporary humans have shifted to living indoors with electricity, man-made artificial lighting systems, and restricted solar exposure. As a result, we have created light deficits and toxins that significantly influence our health and survival.

Some people have calculated the difference in light exposure between living outside and living inside, claiming that the difference is around 1000-fold, and in many cases, so much more. What are the health consequences? You may already be aware of the most prevalent light-related health issues: vitamin D insufficiency (caused by insufficient UV radiation) and circadian rhythm disturbance (caused by excessive exposure to blue-enriched light).

These two light-related health concerns alone account for a significant burden of sickness in the modern world. These two problems, however, are only the tip of the iceberg when it comes to light-related diseases, despite being related to different forms of cancer, heart disease, obesity, diabetes, neurological illness, and a host of other disorders. In the same way, our contemporary world of processed foods leads to severe malnutrition, our modern light environment (with artificial lighting) is a starvation of light or mal-illumination.

Too many people in the modern world suffer from chronic mal-illumination and are unfortunately unaware of it. This problem has far-reaching consequences for our brain and organ function, immune system, energy levels, mood, neurotransmitter balance, and hormone levels. Sunlight deficiency is directly related to anemia, depression, fat mass in the body, and digestive problems.

Artificial lighting has become such a huge problem in our modern world that many researchers call it "light pollution" in a way that would not have been possible even 10 years ago. Artificial light source pollution seriously impacts the quality of life for both people and animals and is potentially causing the degradation of our environment through eutrophication much more rapidly than previously thought.

But what if I told you there is another type of light shortage that most people are completely ignorant of and that is likely far more dangerous? A lack of red and near-infrared (NIR) light. In terms of human health, the red and near-infrared portions of the light spectrum are the most fascinating and potent. They are associated with most of our body's natural rhythms and the production of nighttime melatonin. They also influence the health of our brain, skin, and eyes.

You'll be blown away when you understand what these types of light can accomplish inside our bodies—specifically, how our cells use them to make more energy—and how they are responsible for tissue regeneration, repair, and healthy inflammation pathways in our body. You'll be shocked at how many diseases we suffer from could be prevented by increasing our body's exposure to these light waves and what the research has to say about it. So, what do red and NIR light have to do with each other? Aren't they technically different? Let's find out.

Red Light and Near-Infrared Light

21

Some might say that it's like comparing the Lion to the Lamb, but it just might surprise you that both types of light have unique properties and applications. While red light falls within the visible spectrum and is commonly associated with warmth and energy, near-infrared light lies just beyond the red end of the spectrum and possesses its own set of intriguing characteristics. Understanding the differences between these two types of light can shed light on their diverse uses in various fields, ranging from medicine to agriculture to beauty.

The spectrum of light is a continuous series reaching from long wavelengths, such as radio and microwaves, to short wavelengths, such as gamma rays and X-rays. When we add up all the light waves within the visible spectrum (380 nanometers to 760 nanometers), we get a band that encompasses the reds, oranges, and yellows on one side; the greens, blues, and violets on the other; and everything in between. Red light represents the longest wavelengths in this visible light spectrum and is commonly associated with the sun and other decorative colors (think fire engines) because of its warmth. On the other hand, near-infrared light has wavelengths that are longer than red light but shorter than far-infrared light. Humans have been able to produce both types of light throughout history by utilizing different techniques like incandescent lamps or lasers.

While near-infrared lies just outside the visible spectrum, it is directly adjacent to it and can be perceived by its effect on objects that are sensitive to it. A good example of this is a camera's auto-focus function. While we don't notice the light, our camera lenses are able to distinguish near-infrared light from objects in the distance, allowing the lens to adjust its focus accordingly. Similarly, infrared cameras can see humans and animals in the dark because the surrounding undetectable near-infrared light readily absorbs the heat emitted by our bodies.

The real question, however, is: why are these two types of light used the way they are? To answer this, we must first understand what light can do and how it's transferred.

When talking about light, scientists refer to it as the visible spectrum, electromagnetic energy, and a photon (or wave). As a wave, it can travel through the air and space. When applied to our skin at various wavelengths, it can penetrate the dermal layer through our skin's pigment molecules. Once in the bloodstream or lymph system, this energy has access to our cells.

So, what does this mean? It means that the light wave, with its energy and photons, can now penetrate our cell membranes and enter our living, complex biological system. Once inside, the light waves can interact with the cell's proteins, DNA, and other biomolecules to affect its functioning.

At this point, we've established how light waves can transfer their energy into the bloodstream and cells; however, another big question remains unanswered. What is the difference between red light and near-infrared light?

Red Light vs. Near-Infrared Light: What's the Difference?

As you might guess, some key differences between red and near-infrared light exist. Let's take a closer look.

Red light has the longest wavelengths within the visible spectrum. This means that it's capable of penetrating our skin to the deepest and stimulating the largest cells, such as bone marrow and fibroblasts. If you think about it, red light has a very active life compared to other wavelengths in the visible spectrum. Red is typically associated with fire, and its long wavelength makes it ideal for heating things up. It is also used to speed up chemical reactions, making it the primary light used in industrial settings to regulate chemical reactions and speed them up.

On the other hand, near-infrared light has wavelengths longer than red light but shorter than far-infrared light. While both substances have a long wavelength, near-infrared is considerably longer. Near-infrared's wavelength is 760 to 2,000 nanometers, which is close to what red light has but not quite. Its longer wavelength makes it ideal for penetrating deeper into our bodies, with less light being absorbed by skin pigments and tissues. While red light can be used to activate cytochrome c oxidase, the enzyme responsible for producing energy in living cells and healing wounds, near-infrared light is capable of interacting with nearly every single biomolecule within our cells. This includes DNA and RNA, proteins, and sugars—all the complex molecules within a cell that give it structure.

When it comes to using near-infrared light on the body, this is one type of light that you cannot see with your naked eye. In fact, if you stare at a near-infrared lamp, you will see nothing but darkness. Nonetheless, regardless of its invisibility, recent studies have suggested that near-infrared light can be an effective treatment in ways similar to red light therapy. Both types of light can work as antioxidants, stimulate blood flow, and eliminate harmful bacteria and viruses because they're both composed of photons (energy) and have the ability to penetrate the skin's dermal layer.

Researchers have also found that near-infrared penetrates more deeply into the skin and stimulates the blood flow required for healthy cell metabolism, making it a very effective method of treating skin disorders like acne, eczema, and psoriasis.

Red Light Therapy vs. Near-Infrared Therapy

While both red and near-infrared light therapy are effective treatments for skin issues and cell metabolism, there are some differences in how they work.

Red light promotes collagen production associated with the skin's dermal layer. Not only does it stimulate new collagen formation, but it also helps expedite the healing process when used as a treatment for scar tissue and skin irritations like acne. As a result, red light is the go-to treatment for any skin conditions that require collagen production to aid in healing, like rosacea and eczema, as well as wounds and scar tissue.

In contrast, near-infrared light appears to be more effective at increasing blood flow within the dermis layer of the skin. This keeps the skin smooth and the pores tighter to prevent water loss, which is a cause of wrinkles. Near-infrared light has similar properties to red light, but its wavelengths are more suitable for vascular tissue and blood vessels within the skin.

Another important difference between red and near-infrared light therapy is how they affect the body's internal systems. While red light has the longest wavelength within the visible spectrum, near-infrared is adjacent to red and can penetrate deeper into the skin due to its much longer wavelength. These differences in penetration depth and targeted areas make red light therapy more preferred for surface-level skin concerns like acne and sun damage, while near-infrared therapy is often used for more severe conditions like wounds and deep tissue injuries. Additionally, red light therapy is generally considered to be a non-invasive and gentle treatment, while near-infrared therapy may cause a slight warming sensation due to its deeper penetration.

In addition to these two specific differences, there is also a tremendous amount of research that has been conducted regarding red light therapy. In contrast, there is no long-term research on the effects of near-infrared light therapy. As a consequence, its true potential as an effective treatment method remains unclear at the moment. Researchers hope to find new and exciting ways to use near-infrared light therapy for many medical conditions, but for now, red light therapy is the treatment of choice for a plethora of health conditions. These differences between red and near-infrared light will continue to spark debates about their effectiveness in the medical realm, especially since they are so similar in their properties.

Similarities between Red Light Therapy and Near-Infrared Therapy

1. Both treatments increase blood flow

Blood flow is the life force of the body and essential for cell metabolism, especially when it comes to repairing damaged tissues. Red light therapy can increase blood flow by as much as 10% within a few minutes of exposure, while near-infrared therapy has been shown to significantly improve blood circulation throughout the body. Additionally, both treatments have been found to promote the production of nitric oxide, a molecule that helps relax and widen blood vessels, further enhancing blood flow. These improvements in blood circulation can have a multitude of benefits for your health and well-being. One of the main advantages is the ability to deliver oxygen and nutrients more efficiently to different parts of the body, aiding in the healing process and reducing inflammation. This can be particularly beneficial for anyone recovering from injuries or surgeries because it can accelerate the regeneration of tissues and promote faster healing. Furthermore, enhanced blood flow can also help remove waste products and toxins from the body, improving detoxification and overall cellular function.

2. Both treatments have antioxidant properties

Antioxidants are powerful free radical scavengers that have been shown to protect the body against many different ailments. Both red and near-infrared light treatments have been found to have antioxidant properties and can stimulate the production of glutathione, an important antioxidant that helps neutralize harmful free radicals. Another similar effect is the stimulation of superoxide dismutase (SOD), a type of enzyme that also helps block free radicals from damaging healthy cells.

3. Both treatments have anti-inflammatory effects

Inflammation is a natural immune response to infection or injury but is also a primary factor in many chronic diseases. Red light therapy has been shown to suppress the production of pro-inflammatory cytokines like TNF-α as well as other enzymes associated with inflammation. In fact, research shows that red light treatment is comparable to corticosteroid drug treatment for inflammation and pain relief. On top of its anti-inflammatory properties, red light therapy has also been found to stimulate the production of interleukin-10 (IL-10), another anti-inflammatory molecule that can reduce the severity and duration of inflammation. On the other hand, near-infrared light therapy has also been found to have powerful anti-inflammatory effects. It can reduce pro-inflammatory cytokines like IL-1b and has been reported to stimulate the production of IL-10 in mice. There is also evidence that near-infrared light therapy may be useful for treating acne, and studies have shown that it may be as effective as conventional treatments in preventing recurrence and improving existing acne scarring.

4. Both treatments have been found to increase the production of collagen

Collagen is a fibrous protein that is essential for maintaining healthy skin and joints and plays a critical role in tissue regeneration and repair. Due to the proliferation of collagen fibers within the body, collagen plays a vital role in tissue repair and regeneration. Both red light therapy and near-infrared light therapy have been shown to increase the production of collagen within skin, muscles, and joints, as well as bone tissue.

5. Both treatments are beneficial for bone health

Bone is rapidly becoming recognized as one of the most important parts of our body since it provides structural support for almost every other organ in our bodies. Bone health is essential for preventing bone-related diseases like osteoporosis, in which the bones become weaker and more likely to fracture. Both red light therapy and near-infrared light therapy have been found to be beneficial for improving bone mineral density, increasing the strength of brittle bones, and decreasing the incidence of fractures. Research shows that elderly people exposed to near-infrared light therapy on a regular basis have increased bone mineral density as well as increased physical strength.

6. Both treatments are effective for treating acne

Acne is a common skin condition that affects people of all ages. It is the result of multiple factors, including your genes, hormones, and bacteria. While conventional approaches to treatment typically involve harsh drugs and can be quite slow, both red light therapy and near-infrared light therapy are effective in treating acne with minimal side effects. Red light therapy has been found to decrease pro-inflammatory cytokines involved in the development of acne as well as inhibit the growth of P. acnes bacteria. On the other hand, near-infrared light therapy can be used to treat acne by targeting the inflammatory mediators that cause the symptoms of acne.

7. Both treatments treat eye health

The eyes are extremely sensitive organs with very unique features that put them in a class of their own. Red light therapy has been found to help treat several different eye-related conditions like styes, dry eye syndrome, and glaucoma. On the other hand, near-infrared light therapy in the form of laser therapy is used to treat some different eye-related conditions like cataracts and diabetic retinopathy.

8. Both treatments are used in cancer treatment

Recent advancements and research into near-infrared light therapy can be attributed to its use in the treatment of cancer. Medical studies have shown that red and near-infrared light therapies have powerful anticancer effects and may even be able to halt cell growth altogether. This is especially true for solid tumors like breast, gastric, and lung cancer, which often require removal surgery. Several different types of near-infrared light therapy have been developed for different types of cancer, each with unique properties. Most studies have focused on using near-infrared light therapy to treat skin cancers or cancers of the breast and prostate. However, research in this area is still in its early stages, and many questions remain about the safety and effectiveness of these treatments. Regardless, the future appears promising.

While research is still ongoing, it does appear that both red light therapy and near-infrared light therapy have impressive health benefits and should be used to complement each other. Combining these two treatments will not only help cover a wider area of the body but will also help ensure that you are getting enough exposure to all the beneficial wavelengths of light since they are different frequencies of light. This way, you don't have to worry about any downsides or negative effects of exposing yourself to too much light. Combining red light therapy and near-infrared light therapy will give you the ability to reach all the major organs and body systems, including your circulatory system, immune system, nervous system, and digestive system. This helps ensure that you have a healthier body and that your health is maintained for as long as possible.

Key Takeaways

·   Both red light therapy and near-infrared light therapy have been found to play a variety of different roles in your body. Each treatment has unique properties, including antioxidants, anti-inflammatory effects, vitamin production, and bone health.

·   Dermatologists often use red light therapy, while near-infrared light therapy is often used by ophthalmologists.

·   While both treatments are used for a variety of health issues, they have not yet been compared in clinical trials to see which treatment is more effective.

·   Sunlight exposure is the best source of both red and near-infrared light. The sun-induced therapeutic effects are one reason why people who live in colder climates are at a higher risk for health problems.

·   Treatment with red and near-infrared light therapy is often combined to provide maximum effect, but you must understand the range of different frequencies used in each treatment and how they interact with each other when combined.

Near-infrared light therapy is an exciting new therapy that has a few things going for it. It is inexpensive and does not require a prescription in most areas, making it a great option for people who want to improve their health but don't have the funds or insurance coverage. Red light therapy is also affordable compared to conventional and alternative therapies. As more research is conducted, we can expect to see further studies comparing red light therapy and near-infrared light therapy and further evidence that combining the two treatments is more effective than either alone. However, this does not mean that you shouldn't try both and find out for yourself which treatment works best for you.

CHAPTER 3: BENEFITS OF RED LIGHT THERAPY

"Light is more like the revelation itself than something that reveals."
— Jim Turrell

Today, there is a lot of interest in the potential of red light to treat illness and improve health. We are discovering that red light therapy can positively impact almost every system of the body, even our brains. The ability of light to induce changes in the body has been known for centuries, but it was only recently that this was accurately described and studied. Red light can help you lose inches of body fat, slow the aging process, regrow hair, get more out of your workouts, and reduce pain and inflammation. It can even restore balance to your body's circadian rhythms and improve your sleep quality. There are so many benefits of red light therapy that the list could fill a book, but for this chapter, we will focus on the most well-known ways red light therapy can help your health. People are usually most interested in the benefits of red light for the skin, so we'll start there, but first, let's talk about how and why the skin ages.

Red Light Therapy and Skin Aging

The human body is smart, but it isn't perfect. It takes care of us, but if it didn't have that one big flaw, it wouldn't be human. The body is constantly self-repairing damage as a result of normal wear and tear. This damage includes the loss of our own moisture (salt and water-soluble vitamins), collagen (the major protein found in the skin), and elastin (also found in the skin). But it isn't just routine wear and tear; there are external factors that can accelerate or slow this natural process. One of the main factors is sunlight. When skin is exposed to ultraviolet light from the sun, it produces vitamin D as a natural reaction. But this light can also decrease collagen and elastin by as much as 50 percent in just five to ten years.

There are many other factors that can accelerate the aging process, including genetics, smoking, stress, and diet (high-sugar diets will cause you to lose collagen and elastin twice as fast). While these external factors play a role in skin aging, so does the internal aging of an individual's body. Many of us are aging much faster than our grandparents did due to the toxic environment we live in today. Our skin is exposed to harsh chemicals, heavy metals, and other harmful pollutants on a daily basis. This internal damage doesn't get much attention, but we shouldn't ignore it because it adds up quickly. Here is a partial list of what can contribute to your skin's aging:

1. Free radicals are a normal part of metabolism. They are the result of too many cell reactions in your body. According to Nobel laureate Dr. Elizabeth Blackburn, "Free radicals cause mutations in the DNA that can lead to cancer." These mutations can also contribute to skin aging, which is why free radical damage is so closely associated with wrinkling and aging of the skin.

2. Bacteria, viruses, and fungi can contribute to the aging process by causing inflammation. These external factors are often ignored because we think it will happen to our skin in the end anyway, and we will just have to deal with it. Our immune system is designed to protect us from bacteria and viruses, but this system can also take away our ability to heal. If the entire immune system in your body is overactive, it can be debilitating because your system is constantly on the attack, leading to free radical formation, which again leads to accelerated aging. It is also dangerous to run your immune system in the red zone because it can lead to inflammation of the skin (which we see as skin roughness and sensitivity).

3. An imbalance of electrolytes in your body can accelerate the aging process. Because hormones are responsible for repairing and regenerating collagen when it is damaged by free radicals, an imbalance of electrolytes leads to accelerated aging— especially if you don't eat enough potassium. Potassium is the most abundant mineral in our bodies and is necessary for

proper cell function. It plays a major role in regulating cholesterol, blood pressure, heartbeat, moods, and many other vital functions. The fact is that as we age, we should eat two or three times as much potassium as sodium, and by eating more potassium-rich foods such as bananas, avocados, nuts, and beans (especially black beans), we can lower the risk of high blood pressure because it helps balance the acid-base level in our bodies.

4. The hormones progesterone and estrogen are being produced at a much higher level in women's bodies as they age. These two hormones play a role in skin aging by causing collagen loss.

5. Caffeine, alcohol, sugar, high-fat foods, and certain medications can all inhibit DNA repair and accelerate the aging process.

6. Your body is not able to repair damage from stress as effectively as it does damage from natural wear and tear, so stress-related skin damage worsens with age.

7. Loss of hair and color. As we age, we lose pigment (melanin) in our hair and skin. These pigment cells are responsible for skin color but also smoothness and elasticity. The result is white or gray hair or wrinkled skin. Even if you have excellent genes and take very good care of yourself, you can still have an accelerated aging process simply by losing pigment over time.

The seven factors above are just a partial list of things that can accelerate the aging process in your body. All of them work together to speed up the natural aging process, but what if we could activate our body's repair system, even when it is not working optimally so that it would work at peak efficiency? What if we could protect the body from harmful influences and give it the fuel it needs to repair itself? In other words, what if we could make the body age more slowly? That's a big claim, but red light therapy is proven to do just that.

Red light therapy works beyond your physical appearance because it allows your body to repair all of the damage that causes aging and stress on your skin, hair, muscles, and joint tissues. It expedites the body's healing process and is a cheaper and safer alternative than many anti-aging treatments. But how exactly does it work?

Skin is made up of connective tissue (collagen), which is one of the key components of youthful skin. Collagen also gives structure to the skin and enables it to bounce back after damage. It is an excellent natural anti-aging agent that works by triggering the production of stem cells in the body, which repair and rebuild the skin. When your collagen breaks down due to environmental damage and sun exposure, the connective tissue matrix allows infection to occur in deeper layers of the skin, leading to inflammation that makes wrinkles appear. This loss also causes age spots and fine lines that are natural to aging. Red light therapy increases the production of collagen in your skin by as much as 300 percent and can increase the strength of your collagen by up to 30 percent. It also reduces wrinkles, fine lines, roughness, dark spots, pore size, skin sagging, and even stretch marks.

Red light therapy activates stem cells in the body that naturally produce collagen. It also activates genes that improve skin elasticity and helps to eliminate wrinkles and fine lines by stimulating the body's own production of elastin, a protein that gives the skin its elasticity. By increasing the production of these key components, red light therapy keeps your skin smooth and youthful.

Muscle Damage and Recovery

Your muscles are made of proteins called myoglobin, which are dissolved in your blood. Myoglobin is the main component of muscle tissue and is involved in transporting oxygen from the lungs to the muscles that need it. When myoglobin is exposed to oxygen, it reacts with the oxygen and creates a chemical process called oxidation. Free radicals are produced during this reaction, and they can damage your muscles if they are not neutralized through antioxidant protection.

While protein oxidation is a normal process, this type of oxidation produces enzymes known as oxidases, which in turn produce substances known as free radicals that break down tissue. These free radicals can be the culprit behind muscle damage, and it is a process that accelerates the aging process. The presence of free radicals in muscle tissue will initiate the breakdown of proteins there. You can slow down this process by using red light therapy before, during, and after exercise that causes major muscle damage, such as weight training.

The human body is always trying to heal muscle tissue by using collagen. However, this process often goes awry when free radicals cause damage to myoglobin or muscle cells. Red light therapy can help the body repair damaged muscle tissue by activating stem cells in the skin known as fibroblasts. Fibroblasts are responsible for healing connective tissue and collagen and building muscle mass during exercise and regeneration after injury. Red light therapy works by stimulating the mitochondria in these fibroblasts, increasing their energy production, and promoting faster healing of muscle tissue.

Red light also acts on the cytosol. In every cell, there is a substance called the cytosol. This substance surrounds the contents of a cell and is where its DNA, RNA, and proteins are stored. The cytosol contains the cell's protein pump machinery, which keeps these proteins dissolved in water until they are needed at specific sites within the cell. With this machinery switched on, proteins can be made when they are needed and will not be prematurely broken down. This helps control the number of free radicals in your body.

Red Light Therapy and Joint Damage

Your bones are one of the most powerful materials in your body, and they're also active organs that perform several functions to keep you healthy. The human skeleton is made of two types of bone tissue: Compact bone and Cancellous (spongy) bone. Compact bone tissue is found on the outside of bones and is what forms the hard outer shell that's visible when you look at your arms or legs. This type of bone is particularly rigid and strong because its fibers are packed tightly together, making it difficult for bacteria to grow there. On the other hand, cancellous (spongy) bone is found on the inside of bones and forms a sponge-like network of interconnected hollow tubes that fill with red bone marrow. The red bone marrow is where all your blood cells are created and where stem cells reside.

As you age, your body produces fewer substances that prevent free radicals from damaging bones and joints than when you were younger. This can cause your bones to become more brittle and susceptible to damage from falls, accidents, or even just the normal wear and tear of aging. Red light therapy helps prevent this from occurring by repairing changes that occur in the molecules of connective tissue. When your bones and joints become damaged, collagen and other proteins are broken down. This generates free radicals, damaging the spine, knees, hips, or ankles and lead to inflammation and pain.

Red light therapy can repair damaged collagen and speed up the repair of connective tissues in your joints, which decreases pain levels. It can also reduce inflammation from overuse injuries, arthritis, or joint pain by boosting T-cell activity in the joints and reducing levels of pro-inflammatory cytokines. All of these benefits help you move more easily and with less pain, guaranteeing a longer and healthier life.

The Process of Weight Gain and Weight Loss

When you put on extra weight, you are storing fat in your cells. The body does this as a protective mechanism in case of a sudden period of famine. Extra fat is essentially stored energy, and it can be used to keep your body running if you are unable to find enough food to eat. However, when the famine is over, and you begin regularly eating again, the fat stays put because your body is not sure when it will be able to store extra energy again.

If you want to lose weight, you must burn more calories than you take in. This concept is simple, but it is easier said than done. This process of losing excess weight is known as caloric restriction and is not easy. It is not only physically difficult, but many people who try to lose weight find that the process can be mentally taxing as well.

Red light therapy has been found to help people lose weight by stimulating key hormones in the body that control appetite and satiety. This therapy increases the body's levels of leptin, which makes you feel full after eating, and reduces ghrelin, a hormone that increases your desire to eat. This will make you more likely to continue your current diet and stick with it long-term, leading to sustainable weight loss.

Red light can also stimulate a receptor known as PPAR-gamma, which influences your metabolism and the release of fat from adipose tissues. Adipose tissue is one of the body's main storage locations for fat. Fat in the adipose tissue can remain there for long periods without being metabolized or used for energy. These fat cells are either one of three types of cells: white adipocytes, brown adipocytes, or beige adipocytes. White and brown adipocytes are used to store energy, while beige adipocytes are used to expend energy. When a certain wavelength of red light stimulates white adipocytes, they are converted into beige adipocytes. Beige cells are a hybrid of white and brown adipocytes, and they make up a relatively new type of fat cell in the body. These cells can increase energy expenditure by up to fivefold upon stimulation, making weight loss more effective and efficient.

Tissue Integrity and Cell Immortality

The cells in your body are constantly dying and being replaced by new ones. This process is known as cellular turnover, and it allows your body to repair itself when it becomes damaged or stressed. It also helps you get bigger, stronger muscles when you exercise. However, as you age, this process becomes less effective. In fact, the rate at which we are able to regenerate new cells begins to diminish once a person reaches middle age.

Red light therapy has been found to increase the rate at which cells are being replaced and the density of the collagen fibers that bind the cells together. This is important because if you are not replacing your dead cells with new ones quickly enough, your body will start breaking down its own tissues. In addition to that, red light therapy can improve circulation all over the body. The more blood that can flow throughout your entire circulatory system, the more cells it can access and repurpose as needed for repair or replacement. This will be particularly appreciated by people who are looking to increase the rate at which they heal from surgery or injury or improve their recovery times between workouts.

Red Light Therapy and Brain Health

Red light therapy is a marvelous tool to help restore and improve brain health by increasing the rate at which your brain can produce new cells. Your brain is composed of billions and billions of cells, but these cells do not remain stable over time. In fact, your brain starts producing fewer new cells as you age. This is because there are certain areas within the brain that stop regenerating new cells after a person reaches middle age. The loss of these new brain cells can lead to conditions such as Alzheimer's disease or other forms of dementia, not counting the less immediate problems like impaired memory and poor mental processing speeds.

Red light maintains the health of your brain through a process called mitophagy. Mitophagy is the process by which old cells are cleaned out, and new cells take their place. When this process does not work properly, it can lead to age-related brain conditions such as neurodegenerative diseases and impaired cognitive function. For younger people, red light can improve their brain health and prevent mental decline related to this loss of cells. The wavelengths in red light have been shown to stimulate the production of new cells in areas of the brain associated with memory, attention, and concentration. This promising treatment can ensure that young adults maintain their cognitive abilities, helping them avoid problems with focus and attention even as they age.

Inflammation and Pain Relief

Inflammation is a natural response within the body when it is injured or stressed. When a part of your body becomes inflamed, blood flow increases to that area, and white blood cells travel to that location to begin removing damaged or dead cells. They also release chemicals called cytokines that can cause swelling, pain, stiffness, and discomfort. This is usually a good thing because it helps your body heal from stress and injury much more quickly.

However, this reaction can become chronic if it lasts longer than is needed. Studies have shown that chronic inflammation might be one of the main causes of heart disease and other circulatory issues. When inflammation happens, a chemical called interleukin-1 kicks into high gear. This chemical causes the cells in your blood vessels to clog up and make them susceptible to free radical damage. It also causes them to behave abnormally, like becoming overactive and sending signals that can lead to pain and inflammation far from where they are needed.

Red light can reduce this inflammation with its ability to increase the production of nitric oxide in your bloodstream. Nitric oxide is a powerful vasodilator that opens your blood vessels and allows more oxygen to reach your tissues. This is what causes you to blush when you are embarrassed. It is also why red light is used in procedures like laser skin tightening. Red light can also prevent interleukin-1 from reaching your blood vessels, thus reducing their susceptibility to damage and their tendency to scattershot blood flow.

Key Takeaways

· Red light therapy can help you lose weight because it increases your metabolism, so you burn more calories daily.

· Your skin can repair itself more effectively when exposed to red light, increasing the rate at which collagen is produced in your body. This helps you feel younger and look younger as well.

· Red light therapy has been shown to improve brain health by reducing inflamed tissues and actually increasing the rate at which neurons are being produced in the brain.

· Red light therapy has been shown to help reduce chronic inflammation throughout the body, which can help maintain a healthy circulatory system.

· Red light therapy is useful for helping you heal and recover faster from sports injuries or surgery.

· Red light therapy can also be used as a form of pain relief when placed on sore muscles after exercise.

The human body is an incredibly complex system that changes in response to the world around it. This change can be good or bad, depending on the interplay between external and internal influences. One of the most important things that you can do for your body is to keep it in constant repair. Improving brain function, metabolism, weight loss, skin repair, and inflammation reduction are all great reasons to use red light therapy as a part of your daily routine. Do not let the flashy, gimmick-like marketing of this product fool you into thinking that it is only for Hollywood celebrities. Red light therapy is a widely proven and highly effective tool that can be used to maintain a healthy body, no matter what your goals may be. Knowing those goals is one thing, but making them a reality is another. In the next chapter, we will go over some of the ways that you can make the most out of your red light therapy treatment. If you are not sure where to start, this will show you.

CHAPTER 4:
OPTIMIZING RED LIGHT THERAPY FOR SPECIFIC GOALS

"As confusion disappears, so does suffering."

— Ringu Tulku

It's exciting to see how much people are embracing red light therapy and exploring its potential benefits for their many health goals. Whether it's for skin rejuvenation, pain relief, or even improving athletic performance, there is a growing interest in red light therapy as a means to achieve specific objectives. With advancements in technology and research, people are now able to tailor their red light therapy sessions to target specific areas or concerns, allowing them to maximize the effectiveness of this non-invasive treatment method. As more studies continue to shed light on the potential applications of red light therapy, it's clear that while it may not be as conventional as other treatments, it does offer a quick, effective form of relaxation and energy stimulation that can be applied to different goals and outcomes.

For example, athletes have started using red light therapy for muscle recovery and to enhance their performance. By targeting specific muscle groups with these wavelengths, they can accelerate their healing process, reduce inflammation, and improve total muscle function. Red light therapy has also shown promising results in the field of skincare. By stimulating collagen production and improving blood circulation, red light can help reduce the appearance of wrinkles, scars, and acne. This targeted approach allows people to meet their specific skincare and performance goals without undergoing invasive, expensive, or lengthy treatments. Like any new technology, however, you must clearly understand what you are working with to ensure you get the most out of your treatment. For that reason, this chapter is about how you can harness your red light therapy sessions to enhance your personal health and performance goals.

Specific Frequency Requirements

Biological systems in the body have evolved to respond most effectively to specific frequencies. These frequency requirements vary between individuals, with some having a higher tolerance for certain frequencies while others may need to avoid certain frequencies. When trying out your new red light unit for the first time, you will want to begin with an initial test run at a low intensity. This helps you determine if the unit is working well enough for you or not. You may notice some slight sensations of warmth and heaviness in the treated area, or you might not feel anything at all.

Knowing your tolerance is important because some people might exhibit adverse reactions to certain frequencies. For instance, certain people might feel uncomfortable sensations in their skin or even experience headaches if a certain range of wavelengths is applied to their face. If you discover your tolerance is not high enough, you may want to tone down the device's intensity and slowly increase it over time. You might also want to consult with an expert and get their opinion before treating yourself with a high frequency that your body might not respond well to.

If you are unsure about where to begin with your red light therapy sessions, feel free to reach out to someone who has been using the treatment for a while. It doesn't hurt to have an expert in your corner, as they can point you in the right direction regarding the best application of red light for your specific health and cosmetic concerns.

A common question that people have when working with red light therapy is, "What frequency should I use?" Research has shown that higher frequencies are more effective than lower frequencies, as they stimulate higher energy output from your cells. However, it is safer to adjust the device accordingly for your comfort level while considering the wavelength range for your particular condition. If you choose a wavelength that is too high for your body to handle, you might experience negative side effects such as nausea, fatigue, and even headaches. On the other hand, a wavelength that is too low will not stimulate the desired effects. For instance, if your goal is to use red light therapy for anti-aging, you may want to target the lower end of the spectrum, as it has been shown to induce collagen production and reduce wrinkles. However, if you plan on using red light therapy in an attempt to boost your athletic performance, you may want to go for higher wavelengths that stimulate faster recovery rates and promote better blood circulation in the muscles.

Maintaining an Optimal Treatment Length

Treatments in this day and age can last anywhere from a few minutes to an hour in total per day. It really all depends on the energy output that you want to achieve from each session. The frequency of your red light sessions depends on your goals and expectations and how long you can dedicate to your treatments. If you want to use red light therapy for anti-aging purposes, you may want to start with shorter treatment lengths without needing a more powerful device. These sessions would not exceed 20 minutes in length. For bodybuilders and athletes who want to enhance their performance, you might find that higher wavelengths and more intense treatments are beneficial to your recovery time. This may mean longer treatment times of up to 30 minutes or more throughout the day. You can also extend or shorten the time of treatment by increasing or decreasing the device intensity level. Red light therapy sessions that last more than 30 minutes might require a lower intensity, while a 15-minute session with a higher intensity may be sufficient for many athletes. Regardless of which method you choose, consistency in your treatment length and intensity is everything.

Red Light Therapy for Acne

Acne is caused when your body produces too much sebum in your skin's pores. This clogs up the hair follicles and causes dead skin cells to pile up. The trapped sebum turns into a breeding ground for bacteria called Propionibacterium acnes, also known as "P. acnes." P. acnes is a common bacterial infection that can cause cysts, scars, and even permanent damage to the surrounding skin tissue. Red light therapy can fix this by reducing the appearance of acne while increasing blood flow and reducing bacteria in the skin's pores. By working to remove bacteria from your pores, you may notice that the redness is reduced, and your skin appears both clearer and brighter.

· **Wavelength:** 630-680nm

· **Duration:** Acne treatment should last 15-20 minutes.

· **How to use:**

You can use red light therapy to treat acne on your face, chest, back, and shoulders. It is recommended to cleanse your skin thoroughly before starting the treatment. Simply position the red light device about 6-12 inches away from the affected area and expose it for the recommended duration. Remember to protect your eyes with goggles specifically designed for red light therapy to prevent any potential damage. Consistency is key when using red light for acne treatment. To achieve optimal results, it is recommended to use the device at least two to three times per week. While doing this, it doesn't hurt to follow a skincare routine that includes gentle cleansing, moisturizing, and the use of non-comedogenic products to enhance the effectiveness of the treatment. As with any skincare regimen, it is always advised to consult with a dermatologist or healthcare professional before incorporating red light therapy into your routine, just to be safe.

Red Light Therapy for Age Spots (Sun Spots)

Age spots, also known as "liver spots," are not a serious medical condition and usually do not require treatment. However, they can be unsightly and can make you self-conscious about the appearance of your skin. The pigment that causes this skin discoloration is called Melanin, which is the same pigment responsible for the color of your skin. A dark brown or black spot may develop when your body produces more melanin than usual. The reason for this unexpected eruption of pigment is not fully understood, but studies have shown that multiple "sun spots" often pop up in areas that experience extreme temperatures. These areas appear as brown or black splotches on the skin. These spots most commonly develop on your face, chest, upper arms, and shoulders but can occur anywhere on the body. Red light therapy can clear any skin discoloration caused by excessive melanin thanks to its ability to increase blood circulation in the affected area, which in turn helps to promote faster cell regeneration in the skin and remove dead skin cells. It also works by improving collagen production in the skin, which helps to firm and brighten the skin.

· **Wavelength:** 660-670 nm

· **Duration:** 15-20 minutes per treatment

· **How to use:**

Like acne treatment, skin discoloration from excessive melanin can be treated on the face, chest, back, and shoulders. Also, like acne treatment, it is recommended that you cleanse your skin before starting the red light therapy session. To achieve the desired results, performing the treatment session two to three times per week for at least a few weeks is best until you get noticeable results. You can also use a combination of red light therapy and other skincare methods to enhance its effectiveness. A topical cream that contains antioxidants after your red light session is a trick that some people use to get faster results, especially since it has been proven that antioxidants can help treat spots and pores.

Red Light Therapy for Anti-Aging and Skin Rejuvenation

People interested in anti-aging treatments are always looking for ways to improve the appearance of their skin. Red light therapy has been shown to help reduce wrinkles and improve skin texture by stimulating the production of collagen. Collagen is a protein found in your skin that helps connect your skin cells together, which ultimately improves smoothness and radiance. Wrinkles are typically caused by sun damage, aging, and hormonal changes, to name a few. As you get older, your collagen production slows down, and you begin to experience the first signs of aging. Red light therapy can help reduce fine lines and wrinkles, improve skin tone, and restore your skin's youthful appearance. The wavelength of light that stimulates collagen production is not strong enough to cause harm or damage, so if you have sensitive skin, you have nothing to worry about.

- **Wavelength**: 620-650nm
- **Duration:** 20 minutes
- **How to use:**

Red light therapy sessions should be performed two to three times per week for at least four weeks to see the best results. Consistency is key when it comes to using red light therapy for anti-aging. By committing to regular sessions, you give your skin the opportunity to fully absorb the benefits and stimulate collagen production. It is recommended to start with a duration of 10 minutes per session, gradually increasing the time as your skin becomes accustomed to the therapy. As always, incorporating a proper skincare routine and protecting the skin from harmful UV rays can further enhance the anti-aging effects of your sessions.

Red Light Therapy for Cellulite

Cellulite is soft tissue distortion in areas such as the thighs and buttocks that causes dimpling or indentation in the skin. Although it is mostly caused by hormonal changes and fat deposition, its cause is still not totally understood. Red light therapy has been found to be beneficial in treating cellulite. It does this by inducing blood circulation in the area and helping to break down fat deposits. Once removed, the affected area becomes tighter and more toned. By increasing circulation and blood flow, red light therapy also helps to reduce swelling and water retention. Add to that the stimulation of collagen and elastin production, which helps to tighten and tone the skin in the affected areas, and you've got yourself a collagenous treatment that is perfect for cellulite.

- **Wavelength**: 660-670 nm
- **Duration:** 15-20 minutes per treatment
- **How to use:**

A red light therapy device can treat cellulite on the buttocks, thighs, and stomach area. It is recommended that you cleanse the area before beginning your session and use 15-20 minutes per treatment at least two to three times per week for one month. A combination of red light therapy with other skincare methods can further improve the results.

Red Light Therapy for Hair Loss

For many people, hair loss can be a traumatic experience. Fortunately, red light therapy has the power to promote hair growth in both men and women. On average, a hair follicle will remain in the growth phase for two years before entering the resting stage for up to three months. Hair loss is generally caused by problems such as hormonal changes, UV radiation, or medical conditions that disrupt this process. Red light therapy can be used to reverse this disruption by stimulating cell growth and new cell production in the hair follicle. This will also improve the quality of the hair that you already have, improving thickness, shine, and texture.

· **Wavelength:** 660-670 nm

· **Duration**: 30 minutes per treatment.

· **How to use:**

Red light therapy for hair loss should be performed on your scalp two to three times per week for a minimum of four weeks. Position the red light therapy device approximately 6 inches away from your scalp and slowly move the device in a circular motion, covering the entire scalp. For even distribution of the light, make sure to spread any hair that is in the way. That way, the red light can still penetrate even the densest areas.

Red Light Therapy for Rosacea

Rosacea is a chronic skin condition that causes redness and inflammation in the face, commonly around the nose, cheeks, chin, and forehead. It is usually long-term, lasting for several years and, in some cases, for decades. It is also more common in women than men. Although the exact cause of Rosacea is unknown, a combination of genetics and environmental factors like sun exposure are thought to play a role. For this reason, red light therapy is tested and trusted to prevent the development and progression of Rosacea symptoms.

· **Wavelength:** 610-650nm

- **Duration**: 20 minutes per session.
- **How to use:**

Red light therapy sessions should be performed two times per week for about six weeks to see the best results. You can also perform daily sessions, but remember that this can be very irritating for some people and may worsen the condition. If you experience any irritation or discomfort during your session, please cut down your frequency to once a week.

Red Light Therapy for Muscle Recovery

Even after a relatively easy workout, your muscles may feel fatigued and sore the next day. The persistent tension and overuse of the muscle tissue may cause inflammation in the area, resulting in pain and tenderness. Red light therapy is effective in relieving muscle soreness after sports and exercise. It has also been shown to accelerate recovery by promoting cell repair and growth in the affected tissues.

- **Wavelength**: 700-850nm
- **Duration:** 30 minutes per session
- **How to use:**

The red light treatment should be used just after working out or training for the best results. Position the device directly over the affected muscle area and leave it on for at least 30 minutes. You can also use a daily 10-minute treatment if you do not have much time, but you still have to do this AFTER the exercise. Your sessions should be performed two to three times per week for up to three months.

Red Light Therapy for Weight Loss

Red light therapy has been found to be effective in helping with weight loss by activating beige adipose tissue (BAT), also known as beige fat. Beige fat has a high concentration of mitochondria, which generates heat and energy in the body. This works to increase the metabolic rate, making it more efficient at burning calories compared to other types of fat. Increased stimulation of BAT can also lead to more regulated blood sugar levels and reduced cholesterol levels. Additionally, it may help control hunger signals by prompting the release of appetite-suppressing hormones.

· **Wavelength:** 660-670 nm

· **Duration:** 15 minutes per session.

· **How to use:**

To use red light therapy for weight loss, it is recommended to expose the targeted areas of the body to the red light for 15 minutes per session. This duration allows for optimal stimulation of BAT and metabolic rate. Consistency and regular sessions can't be emphasized enough if you hope to see results. You should aim for at least three to four sessions per week in combination with a healthy diet and regular exercise, especially if you are looking for long-term effects.

Red Light Therapy for Cognitive Development

Cognitive decline, or the decline of mental abilities with age, is a natural phenomenon that comes as part of human aging. It affects everyone but typically becomes more apparent to you and others after the age of 40 or 50. Although cognitive decline is natural, there are ways to slow down the process. A 2011 study published in "Cell Reports" shows that red light therapy can help promote brain health by increasing neurogenesis (a scientific term for the creation of new neurons) in the hippocampus region of the brain. This has promising implications for the improvement of cognitive function, including concentration, memory, learning ability, and mental acuity.

· **Wavelength**: 650-870 nm

· **Duration:** 30 minutes per session

· **How to use:**

For best results, red light therapy should be performed two to three times a week for the first four weeks. After this initial period, you can reduce your frequency to once per week or even every other week. Simply place the device about 5 inches away from the side of your head and keep it as still as possible. Eye protection is recommended when using this device anywhere near your head because prolonged exposure can permanently damage the eyes.

Red Light Therapy for Pain Relief

Pain is the most common reason that people use red light therapy. It can be from any source and of any type, including chronic pain, muscle pain, joint pain, headaches, arthritis pain, and other issues. Red light therapy has been used to treat all types of pain, from acute to chronic. Studies have also shown that this is a safe and effective treatment option. Although it may not be able to eliminate the source of the pain, it can help by increasing blood flow and oxygen within the affected area. Increased blood flow also helps fight inflammation and will improve circulation and cell repair in the area as well. This can help reduce pain over time if you are consistent with your treatments.

- **Wavelength:** 680-850nm
- **Duration**: 30 minutes per session
- **How to use:**

It is recommended to do an initial treatment every day for two months. After which, you can reduce your treatments to every other day or even once per week. You can also perform treatments as needed whenever you feel discomfort or pain coming on. To use red light therapy for pain relief, you should place the device about 5–10 cm away from the affected area of the body. It may help to perform a session multiple times per day as long as the sessions do not exceed 30 minutes in total.

Key Takeaways

- Red light therapy has been shown to help improve acne, reduce pain, manage weight, promote cell growth in the body, improve neurogenesis in the brain, and provide overall health benefits. Although red light therapy does not work for every condition or situation, it is an inexpensive and safe alternative to potentially harmful medications and surgeries.

- Red light therapy is a completely safe and non-invasive form of photo-stimulation. It takes the place of traditional facial and skin care products, as it is a natural and inexpensive way that skin can regenerate itself.

· Red light therapy can stimulate areas in the body that are not usually affected by other light sources or daytime exposure to sunlight. For example, red lights have been found to stimulate thin layers of beige fat, which boosts metabolic rate to burn calories and fat, reduces inflammation, and improves circulation throughout the body.

· Red light therapy on its own is an effective treatment option for the treatment of skin conditions such as acne, rosacea, eczema, psoriasis, and other skin irritations.

· It can take up to two months before you see results with red light therapy for pain relief, but you should continue the treatment past this time if you see results.

CHAPTER 5: DOSING GUIDE

"In the right light and at the right time, everything is extraordinary."

— Aaron Rose

Ever wanted to know how much red light you should be getting? How long should you spend on your red light therapy sessions? How many minutes are best for different conditions? Well, welcome to our comprehensive dosing guide. There is a lot of misinformation out there about the brightness and duration of red light therapy. Some people think that anything goes; some think you need it for hours on end for it to be effective; others swear by the 20-minute-a-day rule, but what is the truth? You see, everyone is different, and because of this, our response to a certain dosage will also be different. Everything from weight to gender can affect how much light your body absorbs and, thus, how effective it is. So, does this mean that you may not be able to find the right dosage for you?

The answer is NO. There are plenty of successful and happy users who have found their dose through trial and error, as well as more specifically through professional help or by reading about others' experiences.

Think of our guide as a starting point; it's not the be-all-and-end-all. It is to help you get started so that you can then find your own perfect dosage as you go along. Whether you are new to red light therapy or looking to optimize your current treatment plan, this chapter has got you covered and will educate you a great deal faster, so sit tight and let this guide take all of the guesswork out of it for you.

The Importance of Dosage

How much red light you get is going to make a significant difference not only to your end result but also to how you feel during treatment.

Many people believe that because red light therapy is already quite powerful, they don't need to worry about dosage, but dosage is still very important. Red light therapy is so powerful that if you are not careful, you could be putting your body under stress, which can then go on to cause the very symptoms that you were trying to get rid of in the first place. Finding the perfect dosage for red light therapy is an important part of getting the treatment right. Here is why:

1. **The perfect dosage gives you the optimal, most effective results**

Many people find it very difficult to get treatment as often as they would like to. Mostly because they are concerned about how much light they are getting and end up not getting enough of it. The result is that their treatment doesn't go anywhere and often stalls out. You need to find your perfect dosage to ensure that you are giving yourself the best chance of getting results. If you just settle for whatever dosage, you can get away with, then it may not be strong enough.

2. **The perfect dosage prevents the body from being under stress**

Stress is never a good thing in life, and of course, it's not good for red light therapy either. Stress reactions are your body's natural responses to a perceived threat or danger. The stress reaction releases a cascade of hormones in the body, most notably adrenaline, and this ends up increasing your heart rate, blood pressure, and respiration. Another reason why it's important to find your perfect dosage for red light therapy. If you are putting your body under stress, then you are not only hindering your own progress by impacting proper circulation (and therefore reducing effectiveness), but you are also putting yourself at risk of developing problematic symptoms from being overstimulated, such as headaches and insomnia.

3. **The perfect dosage gives you the best results in the least amount of time**

You want results, right? We all do. But you also don't want to waste your time and money on treatments that simply don't work or take too long to give you results. Finding the perfect dosage means that you are able to get the best results in the least amount of time, which is a huge bonus when you are already busy and short on time.

4. The perfect dosage is one that you can stick to

The perfect dosage for red light therapy is one that you can stick to. You need to make sure your treatment schedule fits into your lifestyle; otherwise, you risk falling back into bad habits like drinking too much coffee or eating unhealthy foods. With the right dosage schedule, you are much more likely to stick with it because it's easy and convenient. If you are having problems sticking with the treatment, then you should review your dosage schedule.

Factors That Determine Dosage

So now that we have established the importance of finding your perfect dosage let's look at some of the factors that come into play when determining the perfect dosage for your therapy sessions.

1. Distance between the light source and the body

This is an incredibly important factor in determining the right dosage for red light therapy. Many lights are only effective up to a distance of 12 inches, and some even less. So where did this 12-inch limit come from? Well, it all comes down to the light's wavelength in this case. Obviously, the closer you get to the light source, the more intense it will be and the more light you will be exposed to. The farther away you are, the lower the intensity. However, closer is not always better. Excessive exposure to red light can lead to skin irritation and potential harm to the eyes. Therefore, it is crucial to strike a balance between proximity to the light source and ensuring a safe and effective dosage.

2. Wavelength

The wavelength of the device you use is another important factor in determining the right dosage for red light therapy. The wavelengths used in electronic devices are measured in nanometers (nm), and the amount of nm that you need will depend upon your condition and prescription. Knowing the correct wavelength is crucial to ensuring proper treatment, as it can directly affect both effectiveness and safety. Some devices only emit a portion of their total wattage in the therapeutic wavelengths, while others produce all of their light output in these wavelengths. As a result, non-therapeutic or non-optimal wavelengths may be emitted, which can negatively impact your treatment. This means that you must carefully select a device that emits the appropriate wavelength for your specific condition. More so, an understanding of the proportion of therapeutic wavelengths emitted by a device can help you determine how close you can get to the light source and still be in the zone for maximum benefit.

3. Treatment duration

The treatment duration is another important factor that comes into play when determining the perfect dosage for red light therapy. Depending on the size of the area you are treating and how deep the affected tissue is, treatment duration can vary greatly, from as little as 10 minutes to up to 1 hour. This matters because it can affect both your comfort and the effectiveness of your treatment. Longer treatment durations may be necessary for larger areas or deeper tissue, but they can also be more time-consuming and less convenient for people with busy schedules. The perfect dosage finds a balance between treatment duration and desired outcomes to ensure optimal effectiveness and adherence to the therapy regimen.

4. Treatment frequency

Treatment frequency is yet another important factor. Frequency is determined largely by the size of the area being treated, but it also depends on your condition and tolerance to treatment. Treatment frequencies can range from one treatment per day to up to four treatments per day, depending on the severity of your condition and your doctor's recommendations. As with duration, frequent treatments can be more time-consuming and may make it less convenient for people to adhere to the therapy regimen. On the other hand, attempting to increase the intensity of light in a bid to reduce the frequency of treatments can be counterproductive and may even be dangerous. The correct dosage balances treatment frequency and optimal intensity to ensure effective results without compromising on convenience or safety.

Other Factors That Can Affect Dosage

Sometimes, the dosage you should go with can also depend on your body and unique needs. Here are some of the other factors that can determine the perfect dosage for you:

1. **Age:** The older you are, the more light you will need to get the same results. This is because your body is not as efficient at healing and repairing itself as it was when you were younger. It needs a little extra help to get it where you need it to be.

2. **Gender:** Men and women are not affected in the same way by light treatment. This can be attributed to the different levels of hormones that men and women have. Men are believed to have a much greater sensitivity to light than women, and when it comes to dosage, they might need to be a little bit more careful because there is some evidence to suggest that they are more susceptible to adverse effects.

3. **Health condition:** If you are healthy, you can tolerate more light and, therefore, higher dosages. However, if you are suffering from any underlying health condition, you might be at risk of side effects. When in doubt, it is best to play it safe and err on the side of caution.

4. **Medication:** Some medications are known to increase light sensitivity and may cause an unexpected increase in dosage. Certain medications can also hinder the effects of the therapy. As a result, it is best to take extra precautions when using any kind of medication or supplement that may interact with treatments that use light as a resource.

How Do I Calculate My Red Light Therapy Dosage?

For starters, always remember that you should start slowly. No matter how much red light you want, starting with the lowest possible dosage is advised to see how your body reacts to it. The formula for finding your perfect dosage is not necessarily as complicated as you would think. To begin, you need to:

1. **Determine the light output**: This is the amount of red light your device emits at any given time. It determines the intensity and strength of the light, which in turn determines the potential for harm if it is not calibrated properly. Light output is measured in mW/cm2.

2. **Determine the total treatment duration**: This is the amount of time that you plan on exposing yourself to the light. This would depend on how deep you are attempting to reach into the tissue and how long you want to spend doing it. This is typically measured in seconds.

Now that you have figured out the total light output and the amount of time you plan on using it for, you are ready to determine the dosage that is most appropriate for your needs by using this simple formula:

Total Light Output (mW/cm2) x Total Treatment Duration (in seconds) x 0.001 = Your Recommended Dosage in J/cm2

This will give you a concrete number that you can use to determine whether or not you have achieved the correct dosage for your condition. With red light, you should aim for a dosage somewhere between 3J/cm2 and 70J/cm2. For an example of how this works, consider the following calculations:

· 3J/cm2 is produced by 25mW/cm2 applied for 120 seconds.
· 3J/cm2 is produced by 50mW/cm2 applied for 60 seconds.
· 3J/cm2 is produced by 75mW/cm2 applied for 40 seconds.
· 3J/cm2 is produced by 120mW/cm2 applied for 25 seconds.

This means that if your device has a power output of 120mW/cm2, you should treat a specific part of your body for 25 seconds to 10 minutes (equivalent to around 3 to 70 J/cm2). The same goes for a power output of 75mW/cm2; the treatment duration should be between 40 seconds and 15 minutes (3–70 J/cm2). This leads us to our next topic on the subject of dosage: how to figure out the treatment duration for your condition.

How Long Should I Be Treated For?

The time you plan to treat your condition will largely depend on the depth of the area you are treating. For example, if you are treating a subcutaneous problem like wrinkles, an average dose of about 3 to 15J is recommended, which can be achieved in about 5 minutes or less, depending on the light output of your device. On the other hand, if you are treating a deeper problem, like arthritis, which can be as deep as a couple of centimeters under the skin, you might need to aim for a dosage of 20 to 70J, which could take much longer, again, depending on the device's light output.

To determine the right treatment duration:

1. **For skin conditions**: The skin's thickness is totally dependent on the amount of fat in your body as well as the area that you are treating. For example, if you are treating a small area on your arm and you want to ensure that there is no damage or harm done to any other skin region, it would be best to use a light output of 15mW/cm2 for about 10 minutes. The same goes for a thicker part like your stomach or thighs, where 15mW/cm2 could be used for 10 to 20 minutes.

2. **For deeper problems:** Conditions that require deeper penetration include things like joint pain, edema, fibrosis, cancer, and the like. To treat a more serious problem like this, you would need to aim for a higher dosage. Based on the density of the tissue, you would want to use a light output of 50mW/cm2 for 20 minutes. You could use a 100mW/cm2 for the same amount of time if you wanted to go even deeper.

3. **Other factors that matter**: Things like sensitive regions should be treated with a lower light output than a relatively less sensitive region. Sensitive regions may be more susceptible to adverse reactions or discomfort when exposed to higher light intensities, so it is best to take that into consideration when determining dosage. The size and thickness of the area being treated can also impact the choice of light output and treatment duration. For larger areas or thicker tissues, a higher light output may be necessary to ensure sufficient penetration and effectiveness of the

treatment. However, the duration should be adjusted accordingly to avoid overexposure or potential damage to the surrounding healthy tissues.

Can I Overdose on Red Light?

Yes, you can overdose on red light therapy. Red light therapy is not a treatment that has any significant risks as long as you properly calculate your dosage, but there are certainly possibilities for overexposure. The most common cases of overexposure occur when you use a dosage that is too high and for too long. It's far easier to overdose on superficial conditions (such as the skin) than it is on much deeper problems. Many red light devices can achieve appropriate doses for the skin in a few seconds to a minute. The problem arises when people use these devices two or three times longer than necessary, often under the assumption that doing more is always better. This is a dangerous assumption that can lead to serious side effects like burns or skin irritation. Overdosing is less likely with deeper conditions, especially when the treatment duration is kept to a minimum.

There are many other instances where excessive exposure to something has negative effects on your health. For example, exercise. Exercise is obviously healthy and can have many benefits, but overdoing it can lead to serious damage. The same can be said for sunlight exposure, dieting, and even water consumption. All of these things have some level of benefit, but each has a limit to how much is too much. Red light therapy is not an exception.

How Much Light Is Too Much?

This is not an easy question to answer, as everyone's situation is different. But here is what we do know:

1. If you are having problems sleeping or notice that your heart rate increases after treatment, then this may be too much for you.
2. If you are feeling especially tired or lethargic, then this could be your body telling you that the dosage is way over the top for you.

3. If you feel nauseous and/or dizzy, this could be a sign that you are getting too much light.
4. If your skin feels hot and uncomfortable, this could be a sign that the dosage is too high for you.
5. If you are having any negative reaction to the treatment, then this will not do you any good at all.

The ideal dosage is one that stimulates your body, helping to improve circulation without putting your body under any form of stress. If you find yourself struggling to find the perfect dosage for your condition, then it is highly recommended that you seek out professional help.

Key Takeaways

·   Even though it may seem that the industry has a general consensus on the ideal dosage for red light therapy, there is no precise guideline available. The human body is complex, and so are injuries and diseases. There is no fixed amount of red light that is safe for everyone. It's based on the dosage you use, combined with your own body and historical information on similar cases.

·   Gender is an important variable when determining dosage. Males and females tend to react differently to any kind of light therapy, with men experiencing higher levels of sensitivity.

·   If you want to treat something deep, like arthritis, you'll need to use a higher dosage than if you are treating a superficial issue.

·   The density of the tissues being treated will impact the choice of light output and treatment duration in some cases.

·   Dosage duration should be calculated based on the depth of the tissue being treated.

·   Excessive exposure to high-intensity light can lead to adverse effects.

·   To prevent any form of light intoxication, overexposure, or possible skin burns, always consult a healthcare professional before beginning any treatment. The same goes for using red light devices for purposes other than intended.

Red light therapy is no magic pill. It is not a one-size-fits-all kind of treatment. Red light can be a beneficial form of medical intervention when administered in the right way. It's all about proper dosage, and it can often require more than one session to see the results you are hoping for. That being said, red light therapy is an effective treatment option for some conditions, and there are many cases where it will not be harmful at all. However, the lack of a clear guideline can make it difficult to determine how red light will interact with your body and when it will be appropriate or inappropriate to use. For caution's sake, it may be best to consult an expert or at least an experienced healthcare worker before you commit to a red light therapy regimen. If you're given the green light, you will need a device, and the next chapter is all about red-light devices!

CHAPTER 6: CHOOSING YOUR DEVICE

"The buyer needs a hundred eyes, the seller, not one."

—George Herbert

With more and more people suffering from skin conditions, the demand for red light therapy devices is on the rise. Different models offer different features, and it can be hard to know which one is best for you. In this chapter, we'll focus on the most important factors to consider when selecting a red light therapy device. Whether you want to get rid of acne, reduce wrinkles, or target a specific health condition, there is a red light therapy device designed just for you. We will discuss the types of devices that are currently available on the market, and by looking at the features, how they work, and their limitations, you will know exactly which one is right for you.

Red Light Therapy Devices: An Introduction

A red light therapy device is like a mini-tanning bed but with red light and fewer side effects. These devices aim to penetrate the skin by emitting a low level of red light onto the surface (epidermis), which penetrates as far as the dermis, triggering a process known as photo-biostimulation. In the past, these devices required a professional to set them up, and there were very few of them available. Today, however, they have become more readily obtainable in health and beauty shops.

Every red light therapy company offers a different device with different features, and every person has a different situation, so it is wise to compare the benefits and features of multiple devices to ensure that you can get the best results. Each company offers different levels of intensity for the red light and the type of device they produce, so you will need to consider what you want to achieve and, most importantly, your budget.

Types of Red Light Therapy Devices

Red light therapy devices come in different shapes, sizes, and applications. There are handheld devices that are a bit like a small flashlight. There are also panels that stick onto the walls and doors of your bathroom and bedroom. There are even full-body systems that you stand in or lie down in. The first step when choosing your red light therapy device is determining what you would like to achieve with it and then making the decision based on what suits you best.

Handheld Devices

Handheld red light therapy devices have bright lights that you can carry around with you wherever you go. Because of their small size, they are very portable and easy to pack when traveling. They are useful for targeting a certain area of the body, like the face or hands. These devices are great for minor skin imperfections, such as acne, wrinkles, or dark spots.

Pros of Handheld Devices

· Portable and compact

· Good for targeting a specific area

· Easy to use and convenient for on-the-go treatments

· They often come with adjustable settings, allowing users to customize the intensity of the red light according to their needs

· Are much more affordable than larger systems

Cons of Handheld Devices

· May not cover a large surface area as effectively as larger systems

· May require more time and effort to treat larger areas of the body

· Some handheld devices may have a shorter battery life compared to larger systems, requiring frequent recharging

Specific Applications

· Reducing wrinkles

· Skin rejuvenation

- Acne treatment
- Treating small wounds and burns
- Increasing circulation
- Reducing puffiness and inflammation around the face and eyes

Wall-Mountable devices

Wall-mountable devices are larger than handheld models but smaller than full-body systems. Convenient little panels, they are large enough to cover a wider area but small enough to be moved around. These devices offer many features and benefits that smaller models do not have. For example, they are more powerful, and if they are connected to the mains (like some of the full-body devices), then they don't require charging and can be used for longer periods. Even better, some wall-mounted devices may have an automatic timer, which is great for people who forget to turn the device off. These wall-mounted panels are also usually waterproof and can be used in the shower. However, some do not have a suction cup and must be placed on a flat surface.

Pros of Wall-Mountable Devices

- Larger device that can cover more areas of your body
- Many are adjustable for personalized coverage
- Can be easily moved around so that you can cover multiple skin areas at once, even when traveling
- Generally, more affordable than larger systems
- Can be used in the shower because it is mobile, large enough, and usually waterproof
- More adjustable in the intensity of lighting and coverage of your skin
- Battery life lasts longer than handheld devices

Cons of Wall-Mountable Devices

- For some people, these systems may not fit well into their bathrooms or bedrooms
- Wall-mountable devices require additional assembly time and space

· To purchase a wall-mounted system, you may need to have an electrical outlet available in your room or bathroom where the device will be plugged in

· Cannot cover the entire body with one device

· Some people find them too bulky and inconvenient for some areas of their body

Specific Applications

· Chest or back acne treatment

· Treating larger wounds and burns

· Increasing circulation

· Treating multiple areas of the body in one sitting

· Improving the appearance of cellulite on the thighs and buttocks

· Providing targeted relief for muscle soreness and tension

· Enhancing the effectiveness of skincare products by improving absorption

· Assisting in the management of chronic pain conditions such as arthritis or fibromyalgia

· Offering a convenient hands-free option for self-treatment or relaxation

Full-Body Systems

A full-body system is a great choice for people who want to cover their entire bodies in red light. This system typically covers the head, face, neck, chest, abdomen, back, arms, and legs. By exposing the entire body to red light, users can experience the benefits of this treatment from head to toe. Whether it is reducing the appearance of cellulite, targeting muscle soreness, improving skincare absorption, managing chronic pain, or simply enjoying a hands-free therapy session, a full-body system offers a convenient and effective solution. With its ability to deliver the full spectrum of red light therapy wavelengths to all areas of the body simultaneously, this type of system is perfect for those looking to achieve a deep, comprehensive treatment or those looking to combine sessions for optimal results.

Pros of Full-Body Systems

· Ability to treat multiple areas of the body in one session

· Full body systems provide a more comprehensive treatment than smaller devices

· Red light therapy is well known for its anti-aging benefits, and most full-body systems are excellent at targeting hard-to-reach areas with discolorations

· Very convenient because it doesn't require the user to move from one part of the body to another

· Full body systems are more adjustable in terms of intensity and coverage, so you can easily customize your treatment to your liking

Cons of Full-Body Systems

· Full body systems cost more than the other options

· These systems are almost impossible to pack for travel because they are bulky and large

· They may require more time, energy, and patience for treatment

· Some people may not enjoy the sensation of having red light over their entire body

Specific Applications:

· Reducing cellulite and improving skin texture and tone in problem areas such as the thighs and buttocks

· Treating muscle soreness, joint pain, headaches, and menstrual cramps

· Improving circulation and pain management for people with varicose veins, carpal tunnel syndrome, or plantar fasciitis

· Diminishing wrinkles and age spots in hard-to-reach areas

· Treating hair loss, acne, and rosacea

· Treating chronic soreness and trigger points due to fibromyalgia or arthritis

LED Face Mask

LED face masks are a new and rapidly growing product on the market. Like many anti-aging devices, LED face masks contain red light to stimulate the production of collagen. They use LED technology to emit light that penetrates deeper into the skin to elicit results. Unlike most devices that use LEDs, these masks are designed to target areas such as the forehead, jawline, and chin. This allows for a more focused treatment that can address some of the most common anti-aging concerns and deliver noticeable results.

Pros of LED Face Masks

· The LED face mask is a convenient way to deliver red light therapy to specific problem areas on the face, specifically the forehead, chin, and jawline

· Some LED masks also have additional LEDs that emit yellow or green light for benefits like fighting bacteria or improving inflammation

· Very convenient because you can easily take them with you or use them anywhere

· Some devices also have built-in timers, so you can track how long each treatment lasts

· LED face masks are more affordable than full-body systems

Cons of LED Face Masks

· Like all anti-aging devices, some LED face masks contain blue light therapy, which some people are skeptical about

· Some LED face masks are too simple and do not have the same adjustable features as other systems

· These products are smaller, so they may not be ideal for those looking to treat large areas of the body

· Some LED face masks may be better than others; there is very little regulation or testing on these devices

· The light intensity varies from device to device, making it harder to find a mask that suits your personal preferences

Specific Applications:

· Reducing the appearance of wrinkles and fine lines

· Diminishing age spots and acne scars

· Reducing inflammation due to rosacea or acne

- Reducing the appearance of pores and smoothing out rough skin

Factors to Consider When Choosing a Red Light Therapy Device

When choosing the right red light therapy device for you, there are a few factors worth considering. These include the size of the device and how it will be used, its cost, and its convenience, among other considerations.

· Size of the Device

The size of the device must be considered because you'll want a device that is easy to use. This includes being able to hold it, move it around, and transport it relatively easily. The size is also directly related to the intensity and coverage of light available from a device. Smaller devices, like handheld systems, will typically only cover small areas of the body, whereas larger products, like full-body systems, can cover large regions simultaneously, making them more efficient for treating larger areas or multiple areas at once. The size of the device can also impact its portability and ease of use. A smaller device may be more portable and easier to maneuver, while a larger device may require more space and be less convenient for travel. Ultimately, the size of the device should be chosen based on your specific needs and preferences, balancing factors such as treatment area, portability, and convenience.

· Cost

The cost of red light therapy devices varies depending on the size of the device and what features it offers. For example, a full-body system costs more than a handheld system because it provides more comprehensive coverage in one session. In the same way, devices with additional features, such as adjustable intensity settings or built-in timers, may also come at a higher price. However, before you make any purchase, consider the long-term cost-effectiveness of the device. While a larger upfront investment may seem daunting, if the device provides effective and consistent results, it may save you money in the long run compared to frequent visits to a professional spa or clinic. It is also worth noting that some insurance plans may cover the cost of red light therapy devices if they are prescribed by a healthcare professional for a specific medical condition. Therefore, it might be worth a consultation with a healthcare professional to see if red light therapy is a viable option for you. If it is, researching different brands and models of devices can help you find one that offers the best value for your investment, ensuring that you get the most out of your purchase in terms of both effectiveness and long-term cost savings.

· **Convenience and Mobility**

The ease of mobility and portability is another important consideration when deciding which red light therapy device to buy. For example, some devices are smaller and more compact than others, which makes them more convenient for travel or use at work. Similarly, a full-body system may be better than a handheld system if you want to treat an extensive area of the body, like the legs or arms. However, if cost is your main concern and your goal is to treat smaller areas of the body, like the face or neck, then a handheld device may be all you need.

· **Ease of Use and Adjustability**

The ease of use is another thing you should take into account since red light therapy devices come with different features and settings that can make or break your experience. A device with an adjustable intensity setting, for instance, will allow you to customize the treatment for your specific needs. This is particularly useful if you have sensitive skin or are treating a condition, like acne or rosacea, that requires a certain light intensity to be safe yet effective. Likewise, a device that has built-in timers and automatic shut-off will allow you to easily choose how long you want to use the device for, which can help you track your progress while still maintaining a regimen for best results.

· **Light Intensity**

Light intensity is crucial to consider when choosing which red light therapy device is best for you. The intensity of the light emitted is not only related to the type of treatment you will be doing—whether that be a full-body system or a handheld system—but also to how much light actually penetrates the skin. The intensity of the light that comes out of the device should be high enough to be effective yet low enough to avoid overexposure and irritation. It is critical to strike a balance between a light intensity that provides the desired therapeutic benefits and one that is not harmful. Furthermore, different people may have varying levels of light sensitivity, so what works for one person may not necessarily work for another, so consider your own skin type and tolerance for light when making your selection.

· **Treatment Area Coverage**

Coverage is another crucial factor to consider. Each device varies in how much skin it covers, with some covering more than others. In general, some handheld devices may only be able to treat very small areas of the body, whereas larger devices like LED panels can cover more regions of the body in one session. This is particularly helpful if you have multiple areas that need treatment at once or want to treat a large area, such as the back. However, if you are looking to treat a smaller area that is relatively easy to reach, a smaller device may be easier to maneuver.

· **RFE and EMF Protection**

For some people, RFE and/or EMF protection is a must-have feature when choosing their red light therapy device. RFE and EMF protection refers to the ability of the device to shield against radio-frequency electromagnetic fields, which can leak out of the device. Although devices with RFE and/or EMF protection typically cost a bit more, if you have sensitive skin or have had any adverse reactions to red light devices in the past, it may be worth investing in protective features that allow you to use your device without having negative reactions.

· **Device Durability and Warranty**

Just like with any other piece of equipment, red light therapy devices are likely to break at some point, but the key is to buy from a company that offers a solid warranty and reliable customer service for the duration of your device's lifespan. Otherwise, you'll be stuck paying for costly repairs, which can quickly add up to a hefty price. Even worse, if your company is not receptive to customer service inquiries or refuses to replace a faulty product, you are left without a working device and without options unless you purchase another device from another manufacturer. A good rule of thumb is to always purchase from a reputable and well-established company with an impressive customer service track record and an existing customer satisfaction rating. Customer reviews can really save the day here. It's also helpful to see what others are saying about certain features, such as the intensity of the lights, ease of mobility, and treatment area coverage.

A quality red light therapy device is a product that offers strong, consistent results while also being affordable. Yet, just like with all products, there are different levels of quality and value available depending on what features you want and what benefits they provide. This guide is simply a comprehensive breakdown of what to look for in a red light therapy device, but it is not meant to be a definitive list. Depending on the type of device you are interested in, certain features may not be as important as others, so it is best to do some research before making your final decision on how to spend your bucks.

Key Takeaways

·   Make sure to choose a reputable brand with an existing customer satisfaction rating.

·   Do some research on the device's features and make sure it is suited for your specific needs.

·   Remember that the value you prefer comes at a cost, and most companies offer varying levels of quality and value depending on what features they offer.

·   Do not be afraid to ask questions and ask for more details about the device. Keep in mind that the company you are purchasing from is a business, and businesses want to make a profit.

·   Remember that different people experience different results with red light therapy, so be sure to adjust your own treatment plan according to your needs.

·   Consider purchasing an RFE and EMF-protected device if you have sensitive skin or are prone to having negative reactions to other devices.

·   A good red light therapy device is one that provides consistent results, which you will notice from day one.

·   Size matters! The bigger the device, the more skin it can treat in one session.

·   Finally, if you are unsatisfied with your device once it arrives, reach out to the seller or manufacturer to see what your options are. Remember that they want to keep customers happy, so it is in their best interest to make things right.

Making wise decisions with your money is always the goal when purchasing anything, especially a device that treats your health. Some companies will make claims and promises that may sound too good to be true, and that's when you need to keep a close eye on what you are paying for. Consider a red light therapy device that treats most of your concerns without breaking the bank or sacrificing quality or value. Along with the factors above and keeping in mind your individual skin types and tolerance for light, you should be able to find a red light therapy device that will work perfectly for you and your budget. Now that you've made your big purchase, you will want to draw up a treatment plan that fits into your schedule, and you will need to know all the tips and tricks that will help you get the most out of your new equipment. That leads us to the next point...

CHAPTER 7: INCORPORATING RED LIGHT THERAPY INTO YOUR ROUTINE

"We are what we repeatedly do. Excellence, then, is not an act but a habit."

— Aristotle

With its potential to revolutionize the way you take care of yourself, red light therapy is the treatment of the future. For most, the idea of having treatments done at home without having to go to a doctor's office or hospital and pay for the service makes it seem like a dream come true. It allows for greater flexibility and convenience while also lowering the barriers to receiving treatment. A big plus is that you can virtually administer the treatment to yourself and get it done fast—all without suffering through the hassle of going to the doctor's office. But how do you get started? A schedule.

Creating a Schedule That Works

As with any kind of therapy, the more you use it, the better the results you see. If you want to take full advantage of the benefits of red light therapy, you need to be consistent and commit to a regular schedule. Even if you only have time for a few minutes each day, taking the time to administer your treatments will allow your body to reap the rewards of having more energy and better immunity.

To create an effective schedule, there are a few things you can consider:

·   **Duration:** How long will you be using your device?

More isn't always better. What's better is finding the sweet spot between getting enough red light and overdoing it.

· **Frequency:** How often will you use your device?

This is also an important question since you don't want to overdo it or wear yourself out by using your device too frequently. Ease into a red light therapy regimen, and make sure to give yourself adequate rest between sessions. You may also want to take a few days off each week.

· **Setting:** Where will you use your red light therapy device?

The place you choose to use your red light therapy device is important as well. If there are special requirements for the location, such as placement on a window or bedside table, be sure to address these details when setting up your schedule.

· **Time:** Morning sessions? Evening sessions?

You need to make sure that you're using your device at a time when your body is naturally more open and receptive. For some people, that may mean before their morning shower, while others may benefit more from using it while they're in bed at night.

Strategies to Create a Consistent and Effective Therapy Schedule

Red light therapy doesn't require a lot of time or energy, but it does need to be part of your routine if you want to get the most out of it. This isn't surprising since most other forms of self-care require consistency too. You should resist the urge to "wing it" and instead have a set therapy schedule every day or every other day. A successful schedule takes into account your physical needs, your mental needs, and your routine. To create that successful schedule, the tips below should help:

1. Pick a good time to use your red light therapy device

Red light therapy isn't always convenient, so it needs to be used at a time that works for you. Finding a time that fits into your schedule will not only allow you to take advantage of the benefits of red light therapy but also help you stick with your therapy routine. A lot of people are tempted to use their devices for hours a day to make up for their lack of time, but more isn't always better. The importance of frequency lies in how much time you can dedicate to red light therapy each day without wearing yourself out. For some people, this is as little as fifteen minutes a day; for others, it can be twice that amount. Find your ideal time frame, stick to it, and prioritize consistency. Consistency is key when it comes to red light therapy, as it allows your body to adapt and reap the long-term benefits. It's better to have shorter, regular sessions than sporadic, lengthy ones. Experimentation and listening to your body will help you find that optimal time frame. Remember, it's not just about the duration of the sessions but also about the consistency and quality of the light therapy you receive.

2. Seek out a red light therapy device that works for your needs

Not all red light therapy devices are created equal. Choosing the best one for you will help you have the most consistent and effective experience with red light therapy. When selecting a device, factors such as the power output, wavelength range, and coverage area come into play. Higher power output devices may provide more intense and effective therapy, but a wider wavelength range can target a broader range of cellular processes.

3. Build your therapy schedule around other responsibilities

Building your schedule around other responsibilities, like meals and social outings, is another effective way to make sure you stick to it and prioritize your sessions. By incorporating your therapy sessions into your daily routine, you are more likely to consistently engage in the treatment. For example, you can schedule your sessions during a time when you typically have a break or downtime, like before or after meals. This way, you can seamlessly integrate the therapy into your day without feeling overwhelmed or burdened by it. Similarly, planning your sessions around social affairs can ensure that you don't miss out on important events or gatherings while still prioritizing your health and wellness.

4. Don't overdo it

Red light therapy can have many benefits, but moderation is key. Again, more is not always better when it comes to red light therapy.

While it may be tempting to use the therapy for extended periods in hopes of maximizing its effects, overdoing it can actually be counterproductive. Just like with any other form of treatment, your body needs time to rest and recover in between sessions. By sticking to a well-thought-out schedule and not pushing yourself too hard, you can ensure that you're getting the most out of your red light therapy without putting unnecessary strain on your body.

5. Find someone to help

If you're too busy or too tired to stick to your schedule, it may be time to find someone to help you out. Try asking a friend if they would be willing to take over some of your duties and responsibilities while you take care of yourself. If you can, hire an assistant or caretaker to help you with other things. Red light therapy can be demanding and draining, so having someone else assist with the daily minutiae of life can make things easier for you.

6. Get motivated

Eliminating all of your excuses is a great way to get started and stay consistent with red light therapy. Consider an app tracker to help you maintain your daily routine. A lot of people are too busy or overwhelmed to plan their day, but entering the tasks that they want or need to complete on an app will keep them accountable and motivated. Another thing that helps is surrounding yourself with positive affirmations and reminders to keep you motivated. Hang up inspirational quotes or images in your therapy room, or create a vision board that showcases your goals and aspirations. By visualizing your desired outcome and staying focused on your progress, you'll be more inclined to stay committed to your red light therapy routine.

7. Ask for help

If you find it difficult to stick with your sessions, explain your situation to others you trust. Family, friends, or even a professional therapist who has experience in this area could be able to help steer you in the right direction or at least give you some pointers on how to make things easier for yourself. While red light therapy can be beneficial, it does require a lot of dedication and commitment on the part of the individual using it. Ask for help from friends or family if you feel like you lack motivation or don't have the time to take care of yourself.

8. Reward yourself

Another great way to stay motivated is by rewarding yourself for each session you complete. Whether it be a new accessory, a massage, or an indulgence in your favorite food, find something that will help motivate you to keep going in between sessions. The moment you start feeling like your motivation is waning or you are giving in to temptations, give yourself a little reward to keep you on track.

9. Be proactive, not reactive

Proactive red light therapy is all about making your body the best it can be rather than simply fixing problems. If you're proactive about your health and wellness, you'll engage in treatments that will make you feel great, but only in a natural, long-term way. You'll take the treatments that work for you rather than treating symptoms or getting a quick fix to get rid of an issue you don't need to worry about.

10. Patience pays off

Patience is crucial when it comes to red light therapy. Just like in the case of most things, slow and steady wins the race. The effects of red light therapy may not be instantaneous, but they are definitely worth waiting for. While you may not notice dramatic results immediately after a session, the cumulative effect of regular sessions will provide you with deep relaxation and even more motivation.

Monitoring Your Progress

Having the right tools to monitor your progress is essential to using red light therapy effectively. These devices are designed to collect data about your body and can tell you all kinds of things about your wellness and general health. You may be surprised at how much these gadgets can tell you about yourself and the current state of your health and body. There are many different types of these monitors available, including:

1. **Body Fat Analyzer**: This device will measure your body fat with ease. It will also estimate your body weight and your BMI. This is a great way to track your progress and keep yourself motivated, as it will show you how your body is changing with every session.

2. **Blood Pressure Monitors**: These devices are great if you find spikes in your blood pressure when you get anxious. They will tell you exactly how much anxiety is affecting your blood pressure levels and allow you to adjust accordingly.

3. **Heart Rate Monitors**: If you're constantly worrying about your heart health, a heart rate monitor can be invaluable. You can measure your heart rate every day for two weeks or longer and see how it's affected by your sessions, allowing you to take measures to make sure that your heart is as strong as you need it to be.

4. **Sleep Monitors**: If you want to know how your sleep patterns are affected by red light therapy, a sleep monitor is great for you. You can measure how long it takes your body to get to sleep and how much sleep you're actually getting. This will show you exactly what changes are being made in your life by red light therapy and give insight into how your body is responding to the treatments.

5. **Body Temperature Monitors**: As the name suggests, this device monitors the body's temperature. It will show you how your temperature is affected by red light therapy sessions, allowing you to track your progress and adjust accordingly if any changes are necessary.

6. **Electrodiagnostic Device:** This device attaches to the body and monitors every response. It will measure muscle tension and even electrical activity in the body. This is a great tool to use if you want more precise information about how red light therapy affects your entire body rather than just one area.

Adjusting Your Treatment Plan

You may feel like your body has already changed enough to warrant more treatments, but you might be wrong. Your body might have gone through a major transformation when using red light therapy, but this isn't always a sign to up your dose. Sometimes people try to ramp up their treatments without knowing exactly what they're doing, only to find that the results are not as good as they'd hoped. It's a good idea to take some time off from red light therapy if you feel like your body has changed too much or if you're simply not getting the benefits that you expected from using the therapy. Different people have different reactions to red light therapy, and everyone will ultimately have different outcomes. There is no way to know precisely how your body is reacting to the treatments if you only do one session a month.

Red light therapy sessions should not be taken lightly. You are making important changes in your life when you start treating yourself with red light, no matter how little or how much you've done so far. They will change the health of your body and mind for the better, but these changes are not something that can be rushed or underplayed. You need to make sure that you're fully committed to the treatments before you start. If anything seems unclear, take a step back and make sure that you're doing everything correctly. You will know when it's time to up your dose of red light when you feel like your body isn't responding to it anymore. You will also know when you need a break from the treatments by gauging your progress and how your body feels. If you're not sure about either, it's best to err on the side of caution and reach out to a professional or a community of experienced users to get more information.

Tips for Making the Most of Your Red Light Therapy Sessions

1. Don't overwhelm yourself

Red light therapy is meant to be used thoughtfully, and with caution, so you want to take a step back if you feel like your sessions are not getting the results that they should. In this case, it's best to slow down and go through the process at your own pace. Do one session a day, or even just one session for two weeks, before taking things up a few notches. It's easy to try and rush your way through things, but it will ultimately be detrimental to the process because you won't get the best results if you don't give it time.

2. Drink plenty of water

Red light therapy can be quite dehydrating, so it's important to keep up with your water intake. You might need to drink more water than you normally do, so try to remember to stay well-hydrated at all times. You should never go on a red light therapy session when you're feeling like you could use something to drink or even eat. Instead, break up your sessions into shorter intervals and take breaks to hydrate and nourish your body. This will ensure that you get the most out of each session and prevent any potential discomfort or side effects.

3. Stay confident

Maintaining a positive mindset and confidence in the therapy's effectiveness will enhance your experience and potentially yield better results. Remember that red light therapy is a non-invasive and safe treatment backed by scientific research and countless success stories. Trust in the process and have faith in the positive changes it can bring to your life.

4. Keep a journal

Keeping a journal will allow you to shadow your progress and keep track of the changes that you're seeing. It will also allow you to see how you react to red light and what impact it has on specific parts of your body. This way, you can tailor treatments more precisely to the areas that need extra attention.

5. Talk to your doctor

Your doctor will be the best person to talk to before and during red light therapy treatments. They will be able to give you accurate information on the therapy's effectiveness and answer any questions you might have. You will also get advice on a dosage for you that is suitable and tailored based on your body and goals. Your doctor can also give you advice on how often you should continue using the treatment and whether or not you should take any breaks throughout the process.

6. Make changes

It's important to adjust your red light therapy sessions as you go along. Keep in mind that it takes time for the body to adapt and change, so don't expect immediate results. If anything, you should expect the opposite, which is for your body to slowly get used to the treatment and gradually become more responsive over time. You can expect a gradual increase in benefits from each treatment rather than seeing dramatic results during your first session.

7. Take photographs

Taking photographs of your progress is another great way to track the changes that you're seeing and how long it takes for these changes to occur. Different people have different results from the treatments, so it's better to take pictures to make sure that you're getting the results that you want. If anything, this can be enough to keep you motivated and on track throughout the process.

Creating a Dedicated Space for Your Sessions

Setting up a dedicated space for your red light therapy sessions will ensure that you get the most out of each session. You can do this by setting up your lights in any arrangement that works best for your body. Make sure to avoid direct sunlight or anything with fluorescent lights, as these could interfere with the treatment.

You can also set up specific sound conditions, like wearing earplugs and noise-canceling headphones, to block out ambient noise and potentially enhance the benefits of the treatment. The setup doesn't have to be fancy or complicated. It can simply be a normal space where you'd normally relax, like your living room or bedroom. You can even set up a red light therapy chair in the corner of a room, a closet, or an attic. The more time and effort you put into creating this space, the more effective it will be in helping you get from point A to point B on your vision board. A dedicated space can also give you the push that you need to keep going and pursue results, so it's worth investing in a good setup.

Key Takeaways

·   Find your ideal time frame, stick to it, and prioritize consistency

·   By incorporating your therapy sessions into your daily routine, you are more likely to consistently engage in the treatment

·   Consider an app tracker to help you maintain this routine

·   Even if you only have time for a few minutes each day, taking the time to do this is better than nothing

·   It's important to find the sweet spot between getting enough red light and overdoing it

·   Ease into a red light therapy regimen and make sure to give yourself adequate rest between sessions

·   Find ways to make the sessions more fun, like making your own red light therapy chair

·   Don't expect results right away. Results are typically cumulative; it will take time for your body to adjust and show signs of improvement

·   Harness the power of red light therapy by keeping a diligent record of how your session went, what you achieved, and how you feel

·   Get creative and set up a dedicated space for your sessions

·   Try taking photographs of yourself to track progress

·   Give yourself time to allow the treatment to take its course

·   Don't hesitate to contact your doctor if you need to

CHAPTER 8: SAFETY CONSIDERATIONS AND PRECAUTIONS

"It is better to prepare and prevent than it is to repair and repent."

—Ezra Taft Benson

So far, we have discussed the many benefits of red light therapy, but it would be unethical to dismiss any potential dangers that you might experience from the use of this technology. As you know, every treatment option has both benefits and risks, and in our case, the risks are skin sensitivity, eye strain, contraindications to certain medications or conditions, and potential side effects like headaches or nausea.

Despite being an asset to the healthcare industry, red light therapy has been closely scrutinized for its safety risks. It is not just a one-sided, feel-good experience, and it is not without its own safety concerns. Safety is of primary importance in the clinical setting, even when dealing with any "reliable" treatment options, and this includes red light therapy. While red light is generally considered safe when used properly, we must examine its potential complications and how best to address them. The key to getting the most out of red light therapy is to understand its use, follow safety precautions, and consult with a doctor if you have any concerns about the risks or side effects.

One of the main concerns with red light therapy is skin sensitivity. Some people are more sensitive than others, and that's okay, but skin sensitivity is still a concern because red light can cause skin irritation, burning, redness, or a rash that may be concerning for a patient with sensitive skin. Eye strain is another potential risk, as prolonged exposure to the bright red light of a red light therapy device can trigger eyestrain and, in severe cases, eye damage. There is also the matter of contraindications to red light therapy, such as specific medications or medical conditions that may interfere with the treatment or cause complications. All of these concerns are valid and easily avoidable when the proper precautions are taken.

Skin Sensitivity

The first step to avoiding skin sensitivity is to understand what causes it. Red light therapy is not new, but there's still much to be understood about it, so we're going to take this one step at a time. For starters, the skin contains three layers: the epidermis, dermis, and hypodermis. The epidermis is the top layer of skin, with its majority being made up of proteins called keratinocytes. These cells undergo a process called cell differentiation that transforms them from keratinocyte stem cells into hardened layers of dead skin called corneocytes. The extracellular matrix of the dermis works to support and protect the skin's structural components and its outermost layer, the epidermis. It is made up of a loose network of blood vessels, which help regulate the flow of oxygen and nutrients. The hypodermis contains the connective tissue and fat of the skin that help provide structure and insulation from the cold. If you visualize these layers as a stack, you'll see that each layer is made up of different types and amounts of cells.

Skin sensitivity occurs when something causes these layers of skin to be damaged or compromised. When we consider red light therapy, we aim to penetrate these layers of skin to work on internal components, but this process can possibly cause sensitivity in response to the penetration of the red light. If the skin is too sensitive, it will be painful, rough, and red.

There are two ways that treatment can cause skin sensitivity. The first is related to long-term exposure to heat at some wavelengths, and the second is related to the intensity of light exposure. Both heat and intensity can cause damage to your skin and sensitize it by sabotaging the connective tissue and blood vessels, though both are preventable with the proper knowledge and adherence to guidelines.

Not everyone will experience skin sensitivity from light therapy treatments. Factors such as individual skin type, duration, and frequency of treatments, as well as the specific device being used, can all play a role in determining the likelihood of developing skin sensitivity. The distance between the light source and the skin, and even the temperature of the skin, can affect how much heat is transferred to the tissue and how sensitive it becomes.

There's a saying that it is always easier to avoid a problem than it is to fix it. With this in mind, you should take precautionary measures with respect to skin sensitivity and apply them while using red light therapy. Skin sensitivity can easily be avoided by carefully taking the following precautions:

·   Be cautious when using a device that uses high heat, such as the ones that emit infrared wavelengths in the invisible spectrum of light. Infrared wavelengths can reach very high, damaging temperatures and are not always safe for the skin.

·   During the course of treatment, sunscreen is your best friend. Wear UVA and UVB protection daily and limit the amount of time you spend in sunlight.

·   Avoid UV tanning booths for 6 months before and after red light therapy treatments.

·   Limit your exposure to red light devices to less than 30 minutes at a time, and try to space out treatments to limit the amount of time you spend under the red light. It is always better to limit rather than protect yourself against a side effect.

·   Do not use any other light therapies immediately before or after your red light therapy sessions. Your skin can only take so much.

·   Take the time to understand your skin. A good rule of thumb is to never push past mild discomfort. If you feel any burning, itching, or other discomfort, stop the treatment immediately. This may seem like an obvious suggestion, but some people want to believe in the potential of something so much that they disregard their own feelings, and this is a mistake.

·   Maintain a safe distance of at least 6 to 12 inches from the light source.

·   Use a device with adjustable settings. The intensity of red light can vary from device to device, so it's safer to choose a product with settings that can be adjusted.

·   As tempting as it may be, do not fall asleep during your sessions. This can lead to prolonged exposure and a highly elevated risk of skin damage.

·   Always follow the manufacturer's guidelines. Don't push past the limits the manufacturer has set in place for a reason.

Eye Protection

Eye protection is one precautionary measure that should never be overlooked. To understand why, we have to go back to the function of the cornea, which is the transparent outer layer of the eye. The cornea's job is to refract and focus light onto the retina, a light-sensitive layer of tissue that lines the back of the eye and allows us to see things.

Light is a form of energy. When light enters the eye, it hits the retina, which converts it into a form of energy that can be translated into images. Light strikes the cornea and bounces off it before entering this sensitive tissue responsible for vision. The cornea is very delicate, and any disruption in its structure can ruin the eye's ability to see clearly, thus damaging one of our most important senses.

When using red light therapy, your eyes are most vulnerable when there is no barrier between them and the light source. Certain side effects can occur as a result of this exposure. The first of these symptoms is typically discomfort, which can occur within minutes of exposure. The second side effect is eye dryness, which can be equally as problematic as pain for those who use intense wavelengths of red light without eye protection. Dry eyes can lead to stinging, itching, and burning. It is even possible to cause retinal burns from infrared light, and although it is curable, it can still suffice as a good enough reason to never use red light therapy without the proper protection.

Take the time to carefully consider eye protection. Some organizations, like the American Cancer Society, recommend wearing special goggles designed to filter out high levels of light when using red light therapy devices. Other groups and enthusiasts recommend simply wearing regular tinted eyeglasses or sunglasses to protect your eyes from the light.

Both of these approaches have their own set of pros and cons. However, in terms of cost-effectiveness, a good pair of sunglasses is probably your best bet. They can shield your eyes from harmful wavelengths of light, have been proven to provide good eye protection from red light therapy devices, and are inexpensive enough that you won't worry too much if they get damaged or lost. That said, some sunglasses don't do a particularly good job of blocking out infrared rays, so if protection against infrared is a priority for you, it might be worthwhile to look for a pair of specialty goggles designed specifically for infrared light.

In the same vein of caution, some experts say that closing your eyes is enough to keep them safe during your sessions. While this is true, if you intend to self-administer the procedure, you should not rely solely on this precaution. It is recommended that you use eye protection as well to avoid any potential damage.

Contraindications for Red Light Therapy

While red light therapy has what it takes to treat many different conditions, there are still some situations in which it should not be used. The following conditions can make the use of red light therapy potentially dangerous and its effectiveness questionable:

1. **Pregnancy**

There is currently very little information available about the use of red light therapy during pregnancy. The American Cancer Society recommends that red light therapy sessions be avoided during this time, as it is still unclear whether or not a woman's body will be able to tolerate its effects. The impact of red light therapy on a developing embryo is also uncertain and understudied. Some enthusiasts believe that it does not pose a threat to an embryo, while others believe that there is evidence to the contrary and caution against its use. Given the limited research and conflicting opinions, pregnant women need to consult a doctor if they ever want to attempt a red light session. The potential risks and benefits must be carefully weighed, taking into account the person's specific circumstances and medical history. Alternative treatment options can be explored to ensure the comfort and safety of both the mother and the developing baby. As more studies are conducted and more data becomes available, a clearer understanding of the safety and effectiveness of red light therapy during pregnancy may come to light. Until then, prioritize caution and informed decision-making in this delicate situation.

2. Diabetic Retinopathy

Diabetic retinopathy, or "wet" macular degeneration, is a common complication of diabetes that can lead to vision loss and blindness if not detected and treated. While some believe it is possible to treat this type of diabetic eye disease with red light therapy, there is currently no clinical data supporting its use for this specific condition. Anyone with diabetic retinopathy should be wary of these claims and consult a specialist before trying any light therapy treatment. It's even better to follow the recommended treatment options that have been proven effective in managing the disease because, while red light therapy may hold potential in the future, it is better to rely on evidence-based practices to ensure the best possible outcomes for patients.

3. Malignant Tumors

The effectiveness of red light therapy can be hindered by the presence of malignant tumors in the body, as the blood vessels involved in tumor growth can restrict or obstruct blood flow to the treatment area. This can limit the delivery of red light to the affected tissues and potentially reduce its effectiveness. Therefore, in cases where malignant tumors are present, it is safer to prioritize conventional cancer treatments like surgery, chemotherapy, or radiation therapy. These treatments have been extensively studied and proven to be effective in targeting and eliminating cancer cells. While red light therapy has potential benefits for improving quality of life during a cancer diagnosis, it should not be relied upon as the sole treatment for cancer. It is not a substitute for traditional medical interventions that have shown a higher success rate in treating and eradicating cancerous cells. The use of red light therapy in conjunction with these conventional treatments may be explored as a complementary approach, but it should never replace the primary treatment methods.

4. Erectile Dysfunction

While red light therapy has been investigated as a possible treatment method for erectile dysfunction, there is currently not enough clinical data to support its use in this context. The treatments that have been studied and shown to be effective in treating erectile dysfunction typically involve medications, injections, or other invasive procedures. Red light therapy does not typically cause any side effects (unless you are particularly sensitive to light), but it does not appear to be as effective as these conventional treatments either. As such, it should not be used in place of accepted treatments. One small study involving 16 patients showed promising results when using red light therapy on the penile shaft as a treatment for erectile dysfunction. While the results were not conclusive, and there is still much more research to be done, this treatment method may hold promise in the future. For now, however, the best thing to do is to exercise caution with any experimental treatments and make sure that they are safe and effective before putting them into practice.

5. Photosensitivity Disorders

Anyone with photosensitivity disorders may have an increased risk of experiencing side effects from red light therapy due to their increased sensitivity to light. For example, people with polymorphic light eruption (a condition in which the skin becomes itchy and inflamed after exposure to ultraviolet or other types of visible light) may be more likely to experience reactions like increased itchiness or inflammation during or after red light therapy. These individuals need to be assessed and monitored during red light therapy sessions to ensure their safety and best interests. Further studies are needed to explore the potential benefits and risks of red light therapy, specifically for individuals with photosensitivity disorders because this area of research remains relatively understudied. Understanding the specific mechanisms and effects of red light therapy in this population could pave the way for tailored treatment approaches and improved outcomes. Ultimately, the decision of whether or not to use red light therapy should be made based on the patient's medical history and the potential benefits and risks of doing so. If you believe that you are at risk for photosensitivity disorders, speak with your doctor before using red light therapy.

6. Medications

Equally important are the possible interactions between red light therapy and certain medications. While many medications are compatible with red light therapy, some have been shown to have adverse reactions when used in conjunction with red light. For example, a case study involving a patient using isotretinoin (commonly known by its brand name "Accutane") who developed increased sensitivity and swelling of the skin after red light therapy was reported in 2012. This study highlighted the risk of negative side effects when using red light therapy, even in cases where the patient was responding positively to the treatment. It is advised that individuals with prolonged use of isotretinoin or other medications that have been shown to cause photosensitivity should closely monitor their skin for any changes and consult with their doctor if they suspect that these treatments are altering their skin's response to red light. Other medications that have been shown to interact with red light therapy include anti-epileptic drugs, heart medications, oral diabetic medications, steroids, and certain cholesterol-lowering medications.

Side Effects of Red Light Therapy

Even if you are cleared to jump on the red light therapy wagon, there is still a slight chance you may experience some unwanted side effects. Some of these side effects can result directly from the delivery of red light energy, while others can come from factors such as the device being used or the length and frequency of treatment sessions. Below are some of the most common side effects you may experience during your session:

1. Flushing

The reddening or hot feeling a person may feel during red light therapy sessions is a relatively mild and temporary side effect of red light treatment. Some people may also feel a very mild "tingling" sensation during their sessions. This can be mistaken for an allergic reaction, but it is simply the body's reaction to the increased levels of red or infrared light that are emitted during treatments. The intensity and duration of these sensations typically dissipate within five to ten minutes, so there should be no cause for panic.

2. Skin irritation

Skin irritation and rashes are other common side effects of using red light therapy devices, especially between wavelengths of 680 and 900 nanometers, which tend to have higher amounts of the infrared spectrum. You are unlikely to experience this side effect if you are using a device that has a narrower range of wavelengths and a lower infrared output. Skin irritation typically presents as redness and inflammation in certain areas where the light is being applied. These side effects can be uncomfortable, but they typically go away within 48 hours of treatment and should not require medical attention.

3. Photodamage

Regular red light therapy sessions can cause gentle photodamage to the skin, increasing the risk of skin sensitivity and sun damage. This is especially true if you are using red light therapy systems that emit wavelengths between 870 and 980 nanometers. However, the risk of photodamage can be considerably lessened by limiting your treatments to a few minutes per day and making sure that you are using adequate sun protection when you're out in the sun.

4. Headaches

Red light therapy sessions can also be accompanied by headaches, which are typically caused by the wavelengths of light being emitted. Not to worry, these headaches typically go away within a few minutes.

5. Nausea

Another very rare side effect of red light therapy can be nausea, which is sometimes accompanied by vomiting. If you experience nausea after a red light therapy session, it is best to consult with your doctor or healthcare expert to rule out any underlying medical conditions that could be causing this reaction.

6. Dehydration

Dehydration is another possible side effect of using red light therapy, but this occurs more commonly with prolonged exposure to the light. When dehydration does occur, it is common to experience a mild headache and dry mouth. As with headaches, these effects are usually short-lived and should not require medical attention.

Regardless of whether or not these side effects occur, it is better to be aware of the possibility that they may occur during your sessions. Knowing what to expect and how to respond can be the difference between feeling a bit uncomfortable and feeling completely overwhelmed by them. If you do experience any symptoms of side effects, they will typically go away within a few minutes, but prevention is still better than cure. Below are some tips on preventing and coping with these side effects.

· For redness, try applying a light moisturizer or arnica gel after your treatment

· You can apply a cold compress to reduce swelling and inflammation

· Drink plenty of water while using your red light therapy device to avoid dehydration

· Try applying an ice pack or a cold compress to reduce headaches

· Avoid using your device on extra sensitive areas

· Try wearing sunglasses with UV protection while using your device

· Treating the affected area with a topical analgesic gel can help ease the pain

Key Takeaways

·   Red light therapy can typically provide amazing results, although some rare side effects may occur

·   Choose your device according to the wavelength needed and the maximum output of red light energy it disperses

·   Be sure to follow all instructions carefully when using your device during treatment sessions to ensure proper results and avoid side effects

·   Red light can be a safe and effective way to treat a variety of skin conditions, yet it should be used with caution due to its intense energy and the possibility of side effects

·   Red light protection goggles can offer additional safety benefits when using red light therapy

·   Dehydration is a very rare reaction to red light therapy, but it should still be taken seriously and managed accordingly

Red light therapy has its risks and side effects that must be considered and minimized, but its benefits can far outweigh its risks. The side effects that tend to occur are typically mild and short-lived, causing no permanent damage to the skin or body. During your sessions, your main concern shouldn't be whether or not it will cause any side effects. Instead, you should focus on doing what's best for your health and following all instructions to ensure a safe and effective treatment.

CHAPTER 9:
COMBINING RED LIGHT THERAPY WITH OTHER THERAPIES

"A great idea is simply the combination of many good ideas."

— John Maxwell

Do you know what's better than one therapy? TWO therapies! The idea of combining therapies is nothing new. Humanity has been doing it for years. In fact, some would argue that combining therapies is the most holistic approach to healing. The logic is simple: the two therapies can have a synergistic effect, extending the benefits of both treatment modalities by a much larger margin than either would be able to do alone.

Combining therapies encourages us to think outside the box. Light therapy is already a proven treatment that has been around for decades. When we combine it with other therapies, as in the case of infrared saunas, we often find that this can lead to new insights. New treatments are developed, and even better ways of using the old ones are discovered.

The same is true for combining red light therapy with other therapies that are already well-established, like acupuncture. The synergistic effect between the two therapies can result in even higher levels of healing. The good news is that there are plenty of opportunities for you to be a part of this exciting trend. Many studies are being conducted all the time, trying to find new ways to use red light therapy in combination with other therapies.

Red light therapy can be combined with anything from acupuncture, massage, and chiropractic work to more traditional therapies such as saunas and acupressure. Even aromatherapy and vibroacoustic therapy have been combined with red light therapy in some cases. The logic behind this is one of synergy. Both modalities can heighten the effects of the other, with no negative side effects and very few, if any, interactions between the two treatments. As more and more research is conducted, this trend is only going to grow. So, if you'd like to start getting some combination treatment, let's dive right in.

Acupuncture

Who hasn't tried and loved acupuncture? It's an ancient and time-proven technique that has been demonstrated to have profound healing effects on the body. In fact, acupuncture has been used to treat everything from headaches and nausea to insomnia and muscle pain. It's also one of the oldest forms of complementary and alternative medicine.

Acupuncture is a very hands-on therapy and an effective alternative to medication that is often used when the body needs healing the most. It works by sending tiny needles through the skin into the muscle that is being treated. This is done at specific points on the body, which are very precisely determined according to the patient's unique needs. The needles are then left in place for anywhere from a few seconds to 15 minutes. This process stimulates the body's natural healing mechanisms, resulting in increased energy flow to that area. This, in turn, helps with local inflammation, pain management, and even stress reduction. Acupuncture can also trigger the release of adrenaline and endorphins, which make you feel better almost immediately.

In combination with red light therapy, both of these therapies become even more potent and effective. Red light therapy can be used to treat the same problem areas that are targeted by acupuncture needles. Since the light is able to penetrate all the way down to the muscle, it can have a powerful effect on soft tissue injuries, such as tendons and ligaments, or even trigger point release for muscles and joints that are causing pain.

What's even more intriguing is that when combined with red light therapy, acupuncture can be used to treat some conditions that are not normally thought of as acupuncture problems, like high blood pressure, problems in the cardiovascular system, and even skin conditions like acne and eczema. The combination of acupuncture and red light therapy allows for a holistic approach to healing, addressing both the underlying imbalances in the body's energy flow and promoting cellular regeneration and repair. This innovative blend of ancient wisdom and modern technology opens up a world of possibilities for those seeking alternative treatments for their health concerns.

Since it's relatively new in the mainstream, many people are wary of acupuncture, and the idea of having needles stuck in your body might sound scary. You should know that when done by a certified acupuncturist, the risk is low. A trained professional will make sure not to stick the needle in too deep or anywhere near an artery or a major nerve. The needles are sterilized and are very thin to minimize discomfort. Most acupuncture treatments are even safe for children and pregnant women.

Acupressure

Acupressure is similar in many ways to acupuncture, but instead of using needles to stimulate healing energy flow, pressure is applied by hand to specific points on the body. It is a special kind of massage therapy that combines deep pressure and gentle activation of acupressure points. The pressure is applied to the acupressure point using firm, controlled movements that are slow and deliberate. An acupressurist will be able to determine where the pressure points are located on the body according to a patient's unique pattern of pain and tension.

Of all the different forms of healing, acupressure is the one that brings the interaction between mind, body, and spirit to a very fine point. It stimulates Qi, which is life energy. This causes healing to occur naturally by promoting both cell regeneration and organ function. It has been used to treat insomnia and stress, as well as issues like arthritis and joint conditions such as gout. Acupressure can also treat both acute and chronic pain conditions and even sports injuries like sprains and strains. It has proven itself useful and safe, even for psychosomatic, emotional, and mental disorders.

Because acupressure is very hands-on, it's a much more intimate experience than acupuncture and has a different kind of impact on the patient. It is very personal for each patient and addresses the unique pattern of pain and tension that they experience. Combined with red light therapy, some types of acupressure can be very effective in treating chronic pain as well as muscle tension and trigger points. Also, since it's relatively gentle on the body, acupressure is a great addition to your treatment program if you have a lot of pain or tend to heal slowly.

Chiropractic Medicine

Chiropractic medicine is an integrated system of care that involves the treatment of specific joints in the body, coupled with a holistic approach to wellness. Chiropractic medicine focuses on diagnosing and treating disorders of the musculoskeletal system and strives to promote the body's natural ability to heal itself. It is one of the fastest-growing forms of alternative medicine and has been very beneficial in treating issues like back pain, neck pain, shoulder pain, traumatic injuries, and even carpal tunnel syndrome. It is an alternative to traditional medical treatment that uses manipulation and movement to treat disorders in those areas.

When you are being treated by a chiropractor, they will examine the spinal column and use their hands to detect major and minor misalignments of the joints. They will treat the areas of the body where there is pain or dysfunction and apply gentle and specific joint adjustments to realign those areas. The purpose of this is to help get your entire body back into alignment so that your nervous system can function better and you can be healthier.

When combined with red light therapy, chiropractic medicine can be very effective in relieving pain and inflammation. As red light therapy works to target the soft tissue area where the chiropractic adjustment is being performed, it stimulates cellular regeneration and repair, improving the body's ability to heal itself. For many patients, this can mean a higher degree of healing and faster relief from pain.

Cryotherapy

Cryotherapy is another alternative treatment that has gained popularity in recent years. It involves exposing the body to extremely low temperatures for a short period, usually in a specialized chamber. This therapy is believed to have numerous benefits, including reducing inflammation, improving athletic performance, and even boosting mood and energy levels.

Since cryotherapy involves cold temperatures, it can help with pain caused by inflammation. It can also soothe and relax muscles after a workout. For this reason, it is often used in professional sports as an injury treatment (think ice bath) and to help speed recovery time for severe injuries.

When combined with red light therapy, cryotherapy can be a great complement to your health regimen, especially if you are looking to achieve certain aesthetic results, such as improved skin texture or a clearer skin tone.

Electrotherapy

Electrotherapy is a form of treatment that relies on electrodes and electrical impulses to stimulate growth in the cells. It can be used to treat chronic pain by stimulating nerves or muscles, which then trick the brain into stopping the transmission of pain messages. It has also been shown to be effective in treating depression, anxiety, and insomnia.

Electrotherapy is a relatively new healing modality, and there are still many questions about it that need to be answered. There are some promising findings, but the exact mechanisms of electrotherapy on the nervous system remain unclear. That being said, there is still mounting evidence that electrotherapy has benefits in supporting healing and reducing pain, although more research is needed to understand exactly how this works.

As a standalone therapy, this treatment is helpful for chronic pain, but when combined with red light therapy, it can help you recover from injury even faster. It can also help improve joint health, which some patients will appreciate, as red light therapy can be intense on the joints.

Fascial Stretch Therapy (FST)

Fascial stretch therapy (FST) is a type of therapy that targets the connective tissue throughout your body. This tissue, called fascia, courses through every facet of your body and looks like a spider web spanning all the different muscles and organs. It helps to support and stabilize your muscles and joints and also transmits messages throughout your body.

FST has proven to help treat a variety of issues, including back pain, tight muscles and joints, carpal tunnel syndrome, repetitive stress injuries, and more. It also works well for chronic pain patients because it helps restore the normal movement of the joints and muscles.

FST is similar to basic massage therapy, but the difference is that FST treats the root tissue itself instead of the specific joint or muscle that seems to be causing problems. When you have dysfunction in your fascia, it affects the entire body, not just one part. For example, tight muscles or joints lead to a lack of mobility in every other joint and muscle where they're connected. So rather than treating specific muscles or joints, FST focuses on the fascial web, intending to release and strengthen the fascia throughout the body, from head to toe. This is a key component of building health and staying pain-free.

When you combine FST with red light therapy, it can help speed up your recovery from injury and reduce pain. The light helps to target the joints, muscles, and tissues that are connected to the fascia, while FST helps to improve the connective tissue itself. This combination enhances both the therapeutic and aesthetic properties of red light therapy.

Developing a Holistic Treatment Plan

When it comes to alternative pain treatment, the approaches are as different as the people who practice them. Each one is individualized to meet the needs of your body and your lifestyle. Healing begins with identifying which treatments will work best for you and then integrating them into your everyday life. There is no right or wrong way to go about this. You may decide that you want to include all of these treatments, or you may choose a few elements from each category and create your own unique approach.

Either way, the best way to get the most out of each method is by creating a treatment plan that focuses on finding a balance between what you like and don't like about your current lifestyle as well as the methods used to manage your health. This process can be as simple or as complex as you choose, but there are three main components that must be addressed in any effective combination program:

1. Treatment sequencing

In a treatment plan, it is smarter to sequence treatments in a way that works for your personality and lifestyle. Consider what your sleep schedule is, how you feel after exercising, and how much time you can dedicate to self-care over the course of a week. Think about how you want to feel and what will help you get there. Think about the process and not just the results. This can help you prioritize the different modalities that you incorporate into your health program so that you are maximizing your time and getting the most benefit from all of them.

2. Timing of treatments

Timing is important when considering how to use alternative treatments. Treatments should be used at the right time, in the right place, and in the right way. When combining treatments, each will have its pros and cons, and you should consider how they may interact with each other. For example, if you intend to combine both acupuncture and massage therapy into one mega treatment, it may serve you better to schedule the acupuncture session before the massage. Acupuncture helps to unknot the muscles and release tension, creating space for the massage to work. On the other hand, if you schedule the massage before the acupuncture, the manipulation of the muscles during the massage may interfere with the placement of the acupuncture needles. By carefully considering the timing of your treatments, you can guarantee that you are maximizing their benefits and avoiding any potential conflicts.

3. Synergy

A holistic approach starts with a thorough evaluation of your health. Then, you can integrate treatments that are based on the natural principles that are working in your body. As a result, you get the benefits of each treatment while also achieving maximum outcomes from your overall health plan. This is often referred to as synergy because it alludes to the whole being greater than the sum of its parts.

Synergy is possible because when you choose treatments that are based on holistic principles, they work together to help your body heal. For instance, acupuncture can be used to unblock the meridians that carry energy throughout your body. The release of this energy is often the key to relieving pain and restoring balance. By unblocking these meridians, massage therapy can be used to stimulate circulation and increase the flow of nutrients and oxygen throughout the body. The combination of these two treatments can help to balance your body's system by increasing its flexibility and restoring blood flow to the muscles and soft tissue for pain relief.

It is not always possible to achieve synergy, but it is a good goal to strive for in your treatment planning. By using therapies that are all geared towards helping your body heal itself, you can achieve the most benefits from your health program. These three principles can help you "kick start" your healing process and reach your goals of improved health, a good quality of life, and a lower pain level.

As you can see, there are many different ways to work with red light therapy. While no one treatment works for everyone, there are many options to choose from. When you have the right combination of treatments, the benefits can be amazing, to say the least. The best thing you can do is listen to your body and determine what works for you. Determine your goals and how to achieve them. Then, look for treatments that will help you reach these goals. It will also help to check with your doctor before starting any alternative treatment program. They can help you identify which therapies are best for you and can also determine the right approach to guide you on your wellness journey. In the end, it is up to you to decide what options you want to try so that you can feel good, look good, and be well because, after all, your body is your temple.

Key Takeaways

·   Two alternative treatments are better than one

·   Different treatments have different benefits

·   Look for synergistic treatments to make the most of your treatment plan

·   There are three main components to a holistic approach to alternative pain treatment: sequencing, timing, and synergy

·   When combining treatments, be sure to consider both the pros and cons of each of them. This can help you determine which is best for you

·   Always consider your goals when planning your unique treatment plan

·   Always listen to your body; it will tell you what it needs to feel better

·   Reach out to a professional before starting alternative treatment plans

·   Reevaluate your goals and match them with the treatments that will help you achieve them

·   Don't forget that the whole is greater than the sum of its parts

CONCLUSION

In conclusion, Red Light Therapy has proven to be a revolutionary treatment method with a wide range of benefits. From promoting skin rejuvenation and reducing wrinkles to alleviating chronic pain and accelerating wound healing, the potential of this therapy is truly remarkable. As we have explored throughout this book, the science behind Red Light Therapy is solid, and the countless successful researchers who have experienced its transformative effects speak for themselves. It's exciting to think about where this technology could take us in the years to come.

This therapy is already being used successfully in a wide array of situations, and it has the potential to be used even more extensively in the future. As its usage increases, so will our knowledge of it. This, of course, in turn, will make it easier to adapt the therapy to even more cases. When you think about it, there are very few other health solutions with the potential to benefit so many people in so many ways. It's no exaggeration to state that the potential of red light therapy is so vast and promising that it will impact the world in a way very similar to how the internet has. It will revolutionize our understanding of health, wellness, and medical treatment, one person at a time.

Yes, it may cost more than other alternatives at first, but given the track record of success it has had so far, that price is well worth what you are getting out of it. It's easy to take the powers of red light for granted when you are in the middle of experiencing its benefits, but were you ever to stop, you would see just how worthwhile it was. Perhaps it's just a question of time before the world catches up, but either way, red light is here to stay.

REFERENCES

Brown, A., & Jade, M. (2020, February 20). Red Light Therapy: A Complete Beginners Guide for Red Light Treatment: Miracle Medicine for Pain, Fat Loss, Muscle Gain, Anti-Aging, Skin Beauty, Fatigue, and Memory.

Cooper, P. (2000, August 4). The Healing Power of Light: A Comprehensive Guide to the Healing and Transformational Powers of Light. Piatkus Books.

Cooper, P. (2000, June 1). The Healing Power of Light: A Comprehensive Guide to the Healing and Transformational Powers of Light. Piatkus Books.

Danno, K., Mori, N., & Toda, K. I. (1998, March). A new phototherapy with near-infrared light improves wound healing. Journal of Dermatological Science, 16, S230. https://doi.org/10.1016/s0923-1811(98)84374-0

Gale, J. (2018, August 24). Red Light Therapy: The Layman's Guide to Self-Treatment with Red Light Therapy; Learn How to Use the Power of Light.

Mendes, E. (1991). A Possible Explanation of the Unusual Influence of Narrow Band Red Light on Living Cells. LASER THERAPY, 3(4), 187–187. https://doi.org/10.5978/islsm.91-le-01

Mordon, S., & Vignion-Dewalle, A. S. (2019, April 23). Low-irradiance red light compared to conventional red light in photodynamic therapy of actinic keratosis: A way to reduce pain during treatment. Dermatologic Therapy, 32(3). https://doi.org/10.1111/dth.12913

Porges, H. (2020, July 19). Red Light Therapy: How to Use Red and near-Infrared Light Therapy for Anti-Aging, Fat Loss, Muscle Gain, Performance, and Brain Optimization.

Reshetnickov, A. (2014, September 11). The Medicine of Light (Color): Harnessing the Healing Power of Light-Based Therapies to Overcome Cancer, Pre-Cancer, and Other Chronic Diseases.

Sloan, M. (2018, May 8). Red Light Therapy: Miracle Medicine.

Woodbury, F. T. (1924, December 20). THE USE OF INFRA-RED LIGHT THERAPY. JAMA: The Journal of the American Medical Association, 83(25), 2039. https://doi.org/10.1001/jama.1924.02660250077031

Yadav, A., & Gupta, A. (2017, January). Noninvasive red and near-infrared wavelength-induced photobiomodulation: promoting impaired cutaneous wound healing. Photodermatology, Photoimmunology & Photomedicine, 33(1), 4–13. https://doi.org/10.1111/phpp.12282